Go Vegan?

Review of Science

Part 3

By Milos Pokimica

Medical Disclaimer

The information provided in this book is just personal opinion of the author and is not intended nor implied to be a substitute for professional medical advice, diagnosis or treatment. The information provided in this book is for informational purposes only and is not intended to serve as a substitute for the consultation, diagnosis, and/or medical treatment of a qualified physician or healthcare provider.

NEVER DISREGARD PROFESSIONAL MEDICAL ADVICE OR DELAY SEEKING MEDICAL TREATMENT BECAUSE OF SOMETHING YOU HAVE READ ON OR ACCESSED THROUGH THIS BOOK. NEVER APPLY ANY LIFESTYLE CHANGES OR ANY CHANGES AT ALL AS A CONSEQUENCE OF SOMETHING YOU HAVE READ IN THIS BOOK BEFORE CONSULTING LICENCED MEDICAL PRACTITIONER.

In the event of a medical emergency, call a doctor or 911 immediately. This book does not recommend or endorse any specific groups, organizations, tests, physicians, products, procedures, opinions, or other information that may be mentioned inside. Reliance on any information provided by this book is solely at your own risk.

None of the individual contributors, author, nor anyone else connected to this book can take any responsibility for the results or consequences of any attempt to use or adapt any of the information presented inside.

Table of Contents:

Phytochemicals

Earth is a planet. The planet is not just a planet. It is a closed system where balance exists. Balance in nature is also known as a food chain. In the food chain, the top predators are the highest life forms. Beneath them are herbivore animals and beneath them are plants. Plants are the base of our entire ecosystem. It is only the plant kingdom that is producing new energy and only the plant kingdom. All forms of animals including humans are uses that eat already stored forms of energy. If animals eat other animals, they are still consuming the energy that herbivore animals got by eating plants in the first place. However, the plants themselves are not producing as well. They do not produce energy out of thin air. They are just producing biological matter but the source of that energy is actually the Sun. There are some deep-sea communities that instead of the Sun tap into the energy of hydrothermal vents but for the most part, plants are the main producers. It is electromagnetic energy from the Sun that fuels nearly all of the planet's ecosystem. The plants are just creating solid biological matter out of light by the process of photosynthesis. Photo means light and synthesis means creation. Every single protein that bodybuilders will drink from a whey protein shake is made by plants. Everything that exists is just stored solar energy. We are all actually made out of the light. When plants absorb sunlight, they will store that light as chemical energy in the form of sugar or oil. Sugar can be simple sugar like fructose in fruit or some complex form of sugars as carbohydrates. Oil can be also stored as different types but it is just stored solar energy. If we want to live, unlike plants, we have to physically consume some form of energy. Also, we have to consume building blocks of tissue in the form of amino acids and minerals. We cannot use solar energy to live therefore we need to eat. But there is one more difference between animals and plants. Plants cannot move. They cannot defend themselves from animals. If we get too cold or too warm, we will move. If there is a drought, we will move also. Plants, unlike animals, can only defend themselves by chemistry. They don't like to be eaten or attacked and the only way they can protect themselves is by millions of different chemicals that they will produce. Like us, plants too are attacked by bacteria and fungi and like us, they have an immune system to ward off these attackers. They also have an immune system to ward of animals as well so some of them will have extremely toxic substances and will kill any animal that eats them. Plants also suffer from DNA damage by free radicals so they also need to have a defense against oxidation and solar radiation. All of these chemicals are the plant's immune system. Some of them have other metabolic functions as well.

So, by now, the big problem arises for all animals. If animals want to live and want to consume or extract that sugar or fat from plants by consuming them, they will also have to consume all of the other chemicals that are present in the plant also. In nature, food is a package deal. All for the price of one. These chemicals that are present in the tissues of the plants are known as phytochemicals. Phyto meaning plants on ancient Greek. In millions of years of evolution animals that depended on plants for existence adapted at eating some of them. Not all of them, just some. Different types of animals eat different types of plants that they are adapted to by evolution. The reason why we exist today as humans with big brains is the high quality of diet that cooking of hard to digest plant sources enabled. There is no other animal that uses fire. Fire will destroy some of the toxic phytochemicals and will free up the energy reserves in the plants to become more bioavailable and as a consequence, we will be able to digest a wide range of different plant species. It was Homo erectus that was the first one to use fire for cooking. But still, even with modern technology, we are still unable to eat most of the plant's species because of the different toxic phytochemicals in them or we would not be able to digest fiber in them as grazers do. So, evolution still plays a role. Different herbivore species will eat different plants and in time they will adapt their organism to different chemicals that are found in that particular plant. In time adaptation will be so complete that animals would not be able to live without some of the phytochemicals that are produced in the plants that they are eating. In that case, these chemicals would become essential for life as much as sugar or fat are and are known as vitamins. Vita means life. Before vitamins became essential for the life of different species, they were just one more phytochemical. For instance, vitamin C is a good example. In carnivorous species, vitamin C is not a vitamin. The liver of carnivores is able to produce this vitamin because they do not consume it in adequate amounts from animal tissue. On the other hand, humans that eat plant food have a need for dietary vitamin C or we die from scurvy. Vitamin C has become a necessary substance for our existence. Vitamin A, for example, is just orange pigment that we see in pumpkin or carrot. Our body uses beta carotene pigment from carrots to make vitamin A. Before vitamin A became vitamin, it was just a pigment that plants use as a defense against free radical oxidation. It was just one more antioxidant but in time it became an essential vitamin through adaptation. Besides vitamins, there are thousands of different phytochemicals that are not vitamins but are still important to a lesser or higher degree. There was a big debate in the scientific community until the range of experiments was done on the question does all of these thousands of different phytochemicals that are not vitamins still have a biological action in the human body as well.

If plants are stressed and produce some phytochemical as a defensive reaction does that chemical still have a similar role in our organism? And the answer is yes.

For every single plant and for every single phytochemical that exist, every single one has a biological action in the human body. Every single one from thousands of different phytochemicals, and let me write this again, all of the phytochemicals on this planet are biologically active in the human body. This might seem too strange because there are literary thousands of different chemicals that thousands of different plant species produce. Some will have strong reactions some will be mostly extracted without any major impact but to the all practical means, we can say that every single one will have some biological action in the human body. We still have a hard time understanding that plants were here before animals. Animals need plants to sustain themselves and until first plant species evolved there could not be any animal species. In hundreds of millions of years of evolution, the animals coevolved by eating plants. Animals including humans are just "children" of the plants and therefore it is normal for us to have a biological reaction on a wide range of phytochemicals that exist today. We evolved to use these chemicals for our own benefit. Not just vitamins but a wide range of other phytochemicals as well. We still have the capability to utilize, for example, different antioxidants from plants in our own defense or even aspirin. It is a psychological issue for some people. Doctors don't have a problem to prescribe Lovastatin for lowering cholesterol but will have a hard time believing in herbal medicine. In Chinese herbal medicine red yeast rice was a traditional medication for heart disease for thousands of years. But what did they know? Well, it turns out that red yeast contains Lovastatin. Lovastatin was created by the extraction. Most of the drugs today, more than 50 percent of all drugs are extracted as a phytochemical and are not created from zero (Natural products as sources of new drugs over the last 25 years. J Nat Prod. 2007 Mar;70(3):461-77. Epub 2007 Feb 20). In cancer treatment, for example, 73% are not synthetic, with 47% actually being either completely natural products or directly derived from them.

They are just extracted and patented as an extracted chemical and Big Pharma doesn't want people to know this. They like when people believe that drugs are wonders of modern science and not just some extracted chemicals from plants. Taxol, the revolutionary chemotherapy drug, for example, is just literally dried bark scraped from the Pacific yew tree. Until they managed to find a way to grow tree cells in a laboratory to extract that phytochemical, they literally paid people to go and scrap bark from trees. Morphine and other drugs for anesthesia, Quinineand other drugs for malaria, Digoxin, colchicine all are natural. Periwinkle is used as a treatment for childhood leukemia but you would not know that. On the bottle, it would be labeled as vincristine sulfate injection and it is prescribed only medicine. Holistic healers or better known today as quacks in Middle Ages rubbed moldy bread to treat infected wounds. Allopathic doctors of that time that used surgery and bleeding and heavy metals like mercury to "displace" diseases called them idiots that use herbs and moldy bread until a couple of hundred years later when the penicillin was discovered. Allopathic doctors of today still call them quacks but today they just don't tell their patients that most of their medicine is actually herbal essences extracted into a pill with a fake name.

It is the truth that most of those phytochemicals are not vitamins and that we can live without them. They are not essential vitamins but again they are needed because in our normal evolution our body adapted to consume a large amount of those phytochemicals and there will be a lot of health issues if we don't have adequate intake. If we don't take vitamins, we can die but if we, for example, don't have an adequate intake of antioxidants we will not die. We will have higher inflammation that would lead to chronic disease and then we will die from some illness like cancer. Scientists say that phytochemicals are not vitamins but will use them in the treatment for cancer. So, it is a half-truth. They are essential but the effects are chronic and show themselves in the long run. If we don't take adequate levels of vitamins, we could die in a relatively short period but if we are lacking in some other phytochemicals we will "just" shorten our lifespan, have higher inflammation and wide range of other chronic diseases. Then again some of the chronic diseases like cancer can be deadly. The only difference between a vitamin and a phytochemical is not in their origin but in the importance of that chemical to our survival. Vitamin is just a term that scientists use to describe phytochemical that is important to a higher extent to our life.

There are only two vitamins that are not produced by plants. One is vitamin D that we produce ourselves during sunlight exposure and other would-be vitamin B12. If you are a vegan it is only these two vitamins that you will have to supplement. People have an easy time understanding how a shift in our lifestyle has caused the constant and prevailing vitamin D deficiency in most of the population. We have moved away from the sunny climate of Africa where we have been evolving for 60 million years and now, we are in the cold climate of the northern hemisphere with no sunlight and we live indoors and wear fabric to protect ourselves from cold. As a result, we don't have adequate vitamin D levels most of the year and we need to supplement with it. Depending on your weight and sun exposure you should take from 4000 to 5000 I.U. You can take too much of the vitamin D, the upper tolerable level is 100,000 I.U. a day but taking more than 5000 will have little benefit to overall health and can lower vitamin A levels. However, what about vitamin B12? I always receive a question about it. Logic is, if we are evolutionarily adapted to be herbivores how is that there is no B12 in plant foods and only in animal products? The answer is simple. It is not animals or plants that produce this vitamin but a specific type of bacteria. We have that type of bacteria in our colon and we have production of B12 but there is a problem that makes B12 vitamin for us. B12 is produced below the ileum (where B12 is absorbed), so it is not available for absorption. We produce B12 but it is excreted out instead of it being absorbed. In evolutionary terms, it is not a vegan diet that is a problem but an increase in sanitation. In normal conditions, we would drink polluted water and would not be able to wash our hands. Chimpanzees, for example, will touch their feces and later will eat fruit with the same hand. This allows them to obtain B12 on their diets of plant foods. We don't do that anymore and we have sanitation so we do not get enough of that vitamin. We do not get cholera also but the B12 deficiency in vegans is not a consequence of evolutionary incongruent diet but rater evolutionary incongruent environment with clean water. In a couple of studies done on the subject of B12 around half of the vegans were severely deficient and around 20 percent depleted. That is because they don't take B12 supplements. If you are a vegan you have to take B12. Even vegetarians are only 76 percent sufficient (Serum concentrations of vitamin B12 and folate in British male omnivores, vegetarians, and vegans: results from a cross-sectional analysis of the EPIC-Oxford cohort study doi: 10.1038/ejcn.2010.142). B12 is an important vitamin for many functions in the body mainly for nerve and brain functioning and the production of red blood cells. Lack of it might cause anemia and, in most cases, it is not iron deficiency as most vegans think. Also, it will prevent cognitive decline. In people, age 70 about 1 in 5 have cognitive decline without dementia and that will progress to 12 percent full blow dementia and death. Cognitive decline is a loss of brain cells due to aging. This is normal, to some extent. It is not a full-blown cure for Alzheimer's disease but it is a form of prevention. This is because B12 is important in regulating homocysteine levels in the brain. In Alzheimer's patient's level of homocysteine is extremely high. This substance is so damaging that in the autopsies of people who have one rare genetic defect that is causing high homocysteine levels it was shown that it will turn the brain tissue into mush. Even without this genetic defect if there is a nutrient deficiency, the body will not be able to downregulate homocysteine levels creating brain damage in the long run. This is not the cause of Alzheimer's just by itself but it will increase cognitive decline in the regular aging process and having the values above 14 will double the risk of Alzheimer's. In time the brain loss occurs in everyone but in Alzheimer patients, it has a fast and accelerated rate and the logic is that if we slow down the brain loss, we will decrease the risk of Alzheimer's. There are three vitamins that regulate homocysteine levels B12, folate, and B6. In this study (Homocysteine-lowering by B vitamins slows the rate of accelerated brain atrophy in mild cognitive impairment: a randomized controlled trial. doi: 10.1371/journal.pone.0012244) the rate of atrophy in subjects that had homocysteine above 13 μmol/L was 53% lower in the active treatment group that received high-dose of B12, folic acid, and B6. In this Alzheimer study, researchers concluded that supplementation of B vitamins reduced brain atrophy by 7-fold in specific regions attacked by Alzheimer including the medial temporal lobe (Preventing Alzheimer's disease-related gray matter atrophy by B-vitamin treatment. doi: 10.1073/pnas.1301816110). They supplemented subjects with 800mg of folic acid and this is of no benefit because folic acid is not folate. Plants have folate and we use folate but the supplements have folic acid. The human liver, unlike in rats, has the ability to convert folic acid into folate but only 400 mg of it in a day. Taking more than that is useless. Most individuals that are not vegan get enough B12 and B6 but not enough of folate. In contrast, most of the vegans get more folate but do not have any B12 if not supplemented. In this study and in other studies most of the people that have regular meat-eating diet have homocysteine levels of about 11 because they don't eat enough folate that is found predominantly in green leafy vegetables and beans. In America, more than 96 percent of people don't eat even the lowest recommended number for both greens and beans so they are stuck with a homocysteine level of 11 μmol/L. One more reason is fiber. Probiotic bacteria in the gut that feeds on fiber have the ability to produce folate in the colon. For every gram of fiber 2 percent of folate RDA is produced by bacteria. If you eat a minimum of 30 grams of fiber recommended by the RDA you will have 60 percent of folate produced by your own healthy microbiome. Also, when we eat animal products we have an increase in methionine and this is actually a substance that creates homocysteine in the body in the first place. Methionine comes mostly from animal protein. It is an essential amino acid in humans and homocysteine is a byproduct of methionine metabolism. High protein diet, especially a high-quality complete protein diet is responsible for the increase in homocysteine levels in the brain creating brain damage. If you put people on a vegan diet their homocysteine level will drop to 9 in two weeks without any supplements but when we look at long term vegans their homocysteine levels are horrendous. In this study (Plasma total homocysteine status of vegetarians compared with omnivores: a systematic review and meta-analysis. doi: 10.1017/S000711451200520X) vegans had homocysteine levels of 16.41 and vegetarians 13.91 and omnivores 11.03. This is because they didn't supplement with B12. It is one vitamin that is lacking that puts vegans in a really bad situation considering brain atrophy. However, if vegans supplement with B12 they can reap all of the benefits of their diet and then their homocysteine levels will drop below 5. If you don't eat enough fiber and have high protein intake or in other words, you are eating a standard American diet you will have to increase folate consumption. It is one of the most prevalent deficiencies. If we supplement these two vitamins, D and B12, we will have all the nutrients we need if we are eating a vegan diet. Actually, I will correct myself. The vegan diet by itself is just junk. We need to eat organically grown whole food plant-based diet.

Besides vitamins, next in the line of most important phytochemicals are natural pigments. These pigments are created by the plants as a defensive mechanism from free oxygen damage or as a defense from UV radiation. The most important for us is already mentioned orange pigment from carrots and other vegetables know as beta carotene. Our body will convert beta carotene into vitamin A. We are actually one of the species on this planet that is dependent on a plant-based diet and phytochemicals and we will die if we don't eat them. If we don't eat meat, we will have vitamin B12 deficiency in the modern age but if we don't eat plants we will die from scurvy. Most other animals and all of omnivores and carnivores make their own vitamin C. If we look at fossil record, humans in stone age with some meat consumption that was present still had around 130 grams of fiber per day and around 10 times more vitamin C. It is also logical to conclude that if we depend on antioxidants, two of them are vitamins for us, vitamin C and vitamin E, we also depend to some extent on all other antioxidants as well. They might not be vitamins per se but still, we don't have an adequate internal defense mechanism against free radical damage. We need to consume them as well. We did for our whole evolution. All of the other antioxidants and pigments that are not vitamins are still antioxidants and we still need them to a lesser extent.

Without oxygen, there is no life. It is used by mitochondria, through the electron-transport chain to oxidase some specific molecules to create energy in a form of ATP (adenosine triphosphate). Mitochondria was a separate organism in times where there were no multicellular organisms on this planet. Just one more bacteria. The way multicellular organisms developed from a single cellular organism is by symbiosis with mitochondria. It has separate DNA from our own that we inherit from our mothers. We give them nutrients, mitochondria give us energy. During this process, oxygen is reduced to water, producing several oxygen-derived free radicals or reactive oxygen species (ROS) which play an important role in various diseases. Normally, oxygen free-radicals are neutralized by natural antioxidants such as vitamin E, or enzymes such as superoxide dismutase. However, ROS becomes a problem when either a decrease in their removal or their overproduction occurs, resulting in oxidative stress. This stress, and the resultant damage, has been implicated in many diseases. We have mechanism for our own defense against inflammation and free radical damage but because we have been eating an enormous amount of plant antioxidants in our evolution, we must conclude that we still depend on plant antioxidants to defend ourselves from oxidation and DNA damage. If we depend on taking vitamin C, we also depend on taking other antioxidants as well. Medicine does not enforce RDA for antioxidants in general and does not consider them to be essential. I and many other doctors backed by a wide range of scientific studies tend to disagree. It is true that we will not die if we don't eat high amounts of antioxidants, right away that is. But we will still die prematurely. We will have higher inflammation and higher oxidation and that will, in the long run, lead to cancer and a wide range of other diseases and will lower overall health and wellbeing and will shorten our lifespan. Antioxidants are still essential.

There are no phytochemicals and adequate amounts of antioxidants in animal products. On average, plant foods contain more than 30 times more antioxidants than animal-based foods. There is a reason why carnivores create their own vitamin C. Actually, most animals synthesize their own vitamin C. A typical 155-pound goat is capable of producing over 13 grams of ascorbate acid (vitamin C) daily. Goats have an average of 155 pounds and they live in nature and they eat greens all day. When they are under stress goats were able to dramatically increase ascorbic acid production (vitamin C) by as much as 13 times normal levels than when unstressed (Stone 1979). When facing significant health stresses, as a biological defense mechanism ascorbic acid would be created in massive amounts. This could explain why wild animals tend to remain vibrantly healthy until they succumb to old age (Levy 2011). As a comparison, the recommended dietary allowance for humans of vitamin C proposed and used by nutritionists is 90 milligrams. And that is because we have depended on other types of antioxidants from fruit and vegetables as well and because that was in our normal diet. If we compare the average goat to the average human, we can easily see that we are much more exposed to toxins and pollution and much more than in the past. We should be taking more antioxidants today than in the Paleo period and we don't take them at all. Standard American Diet (SAD) is so sad that the number one antioxidant in it is coffee. If we know this, we can see that we are in serious trouble. Most of the calories come from fat, sugar, refined flour, meat, eggs, dairy and where are the antioxidants? Nowhere. And where is inflammation and cancer? Everywhere. Plant food has been so great and large portion of our diet that we didn't have to evolve such a strong defense mechanism against oxidation but that is exactly what is causing us a serious problem today when we have changed our diet completely. Also today, we are exposed to toxic overload from both food and the environment. On the one hand, we lack antioxidants and on another, we are overexposed to mutagens and toxins. Even misguided keto Paleo diet people are still eating more vegetables and have higher antioxidant intake than people on a standard American diet.

Antioxidants are important because they prevent damage to the DNA and also determent the rate of aging. Aging is just oxidation and people don't know this. The element that gives us life, the oxygen, is also the element that gives us death. It is kind of ironic. Oxygen is an extremely reactive substance. Fire cannot burn without it. It reacts to every molecule it can trying to combine with it or to steal its electron. Even metals as iron are not immune to it. Eventually, iron will turn to iron oxide or in other words rust. In normal cellular respiration metabolic reactions will convert biochemical energy from nutrients into adenosine triphosphate (ATP) with the use of oxygen. In 6 minutes of being deprived of oxygen, our brain dies. Even plants that give off oxygen during photosynthesis when there is no Sun, start to take up oxygen from the air and soil to break down sugars to use for energy, just like humans. Respiration is one of the key ways a cell releases chemical energy to fuel cellular activity. But there is no such thing as perfection in nature. Some of that oxygen "escapes" as a free unbound reactive molecule called free radical and then starts to react with all other molecules around it and that leads to cascading of molecular reactions that at the end lead to cellular damage. This damage to DNA is called aging. Because cells get damaged during regular cellular respiration when DNA splits to repair damaged cells its halves telomeres in half. Every time DNA multiplies it halves the ending of the chromosomes that protect the DNA from misfolding. Eventually, there will be no more splitting and repeating of the DNA just damage and death. And the oxygen is to blame beside other toxic substances. The higher the metabolism or in other words the more energy the cells needs in the unit of time, the faster the damage. Small creatures with fast metabolisms are going to live shorter lives than for example giant tortoises with a very slow metabolism that have an average lifespan of 80–150 years.

This effects every living organism including plants. The way that plans defend against this is by creating substances that have one or more extra electrons to give to the oxygen to neutralize the damage. These are known as antioxidants. There is a different array of antioxidants that plant can produce and the most common type in the plant kingdom are plant pigments. These pigments also protect the plant from UV radiation damage besides oxidation. There are two main antioxidants that are also vitamins for us. First is vitamin C that is soluble in water and neutralizes free radicals in water solutions in the body. The second one is vitamin E that is oil soluble (oil and water don't mix) and it goes to the parts that are made out of fat where water-soluble vitamin C cannot and then neutralizes free radicals there. For example, the brain is a "high fat" organ and serious vitamin E deficiency manifests as neuropathy and myopathy, as vitamin E is essential for the development and maintenance of the central nervous system. Vitamin E could prevent lipid oxidation everywhere in the body and without adequate levels of intake health issues will accrue. Beta carotene is also a pigment.

When vitamin C or vitamin E gives away its electron, they become pro radicals themselves. It is important to understand this. There are no, or let say in this manner, very rare types of antioxidants that "just" give electron and don't turn themselves into free radicals. There are some that I will discuss later. When some substance has weak bound to its electron and some more reactive substance like free radical or toxin have a stronger force it will pull that electron away. But still, even that antioxidant that became weak free radical still wants its electron back. The force or reactivity of that newly formed free radical is much less reactive but still, it wants its electron back. Every time we have consumed antioxidants like vitamin C, they will turn into pro radicals in the body. The way our bodies evolved to cope with this is to have different enzymes to neutralize these new substances. The logic behind it is like this: the strongest poison is neutralized, then the weaker one, then at the end the weakest one is removed from the body or neutralized. It is a chemical cascading reaction that lasts for some time until the body removes the toxins or free radicals. If we consumed adequate amounts of antioxidants, they will neutralize the strongest free radicals and then the weaker ones and then down the line, the damage will be minimized. But it takes the enzymatic pathways in the body to do this.

If you just take vitamin E or beta carotene in the extracted form as a supplement you will do yourself more damage than good. This is a reason why some extracted antioxidant pills don't work. You can take as much as vitamin E as you want but that will not neutralize all of the free radicals because there is not enough of other enzymes down the line to take advantage of that unnatural and excessive levels of vitamin E. Most of that vitamin E the body will not be able to remove or utilize in a proper way and that will do damage just by itself. Only whole unprocessed plant food that is naturally full of antioxidants in experimental research showed benefit. In some cases, supplemental antioxidants increased the risk of mortality. Basically, they were worse than just doing nothing and people who take them pay to live shorter lives. In this meta-analysis (Mortality in randomized trials of antioxidant supplements for primary and secondary prevention: systematic review and meta-analysis. JAMA. 2007 Feb 28;297(8):842-57) researchers included 68 randomized trials with 232,606 participants (385 publications). The conclusion was that antioxidant supplements significantly increased mortality. Beta carotene, vitamin A and vitamin E individually or combined, significantly increased mortality but vitamin C and selenium had no significant effect on mortality. But again, we have to be objective here. In most of the trials, they used synthetic vitamin E and beta carotene. There is a molecular difference between natural occurring vitamin E and the molecule that supplement companies create and they do this because natural vitamin E is very expensive to be made. In chemical terms, natural vitamin E is d alpha-tocopherol while synthetic is dl alpha-tocopheryl. When looking for a natural form of vitamin E, always select one that is "d" (not "dl") and the word tocopherol ends with "ol" (not "yl"). In whole food, there are also other types of tocopherols besides alpha that is considered to be a vitamin. There are beta and gamma tocopherols and they have their own specific physiological benefits. Excessive amounts of natural vitamin E might, and I say here might not be that bad as an excessive amount of synthetic vitamin E. Where the real benefit of supplemental vitamin E exists is where you don't have an adequate intake of vitamin E from food. Usually, people who have a standard American diet are vitamin E deficient because vitamin E is found in oils of nuts and seeds in a whole food package. If you extract oil that oil will come into contact with oxygen and then that vitamin E will oxidase or in other words, the oil will become rancid. When you crack open a nut or a seed and eat it immediately you will have the full benefit of natural vitamin E. If you want to supplement and don't eat enough of plant-based oily whole foods then look for a supplement that has naturally extracted mix of different types of tocopherols including both alpha, beta, gamma, and delta types. Some seeds have only one type for example 100 grams of flaxseed have 20.0mg of gamma-tocopherol but only 0.3mg of alpha-tocopherol. If you don't know this you might think that it does not have any vitamin E because it would not be listed that it has on the label. Only alpha type is listed and recognized as a vitamin but that is not a complete picture. Most of the phytochemicals that are not recognized as vitamins will not be listed on any label. Current scientific data suggest that supplementing with a natural mix of tocopherols has benefit if you have vitamin E deficiency and supplementing more than that will have no additional benefit at all and can create problems (No evidence supports vitamin E indiscriminate supplementation. doi: 10.1002/biof.61). The same story is with beta carotene.

There was a line of studies that found a link between lung cancer, particularly in smokers, and cardiovascular disease and supplemental beta-carotene. Why this happens they don't know. So far there is only speculation because that link doesn't exist if beta carotene is eaten in a whole food package. The reasoning is that there might be a range of other phytochemicals in whole food that synergistically work with beta carotene. Individuals who smoke should not take beta-carotene supplements or for that matter, anyone should. Beta carotene deposits itself in fat within the body and in time it can color the skin. Eating too many carrots can actually turn your skin orange. In extreme cases, people will have an orange nose or palms. It's a medical condition known as carotenemia and the condition is generally harmless. But because of the sex appeal people are taking supplemental beta carotene since it is more convenient than to juice carrots every day. There was a line of experiments that found that people who have a small amount or let's say an initial stage of carotenemia have more appealing face to the opposite sex. It is a nice "golden glow" of healthy young skin. This might have been an evolutionary subconscious response to signal the healthy individual with a healthy diet to the opposite sex. That means more chance of a successful pregnancy. It might be a health indicator and this incentive is something that some people are utilizing as a form of supplement to give themselves a nice healthy look. If you want to take supplemental beta carotene then always take the natural form of it and a better option will be to just eat carrots or at least remove the fiber and drink carrot juice. On average, a healthy dosage of beta-carotene is six to eight milligrams a day. According to a Columbia University health blog, "for carotenemia to set in, you might have to consume as much as 20 milligrams per day (or, three large carrots)." Same as vitamin E, in natural whole food there are also alpha, beta and gamma carotenes as well and a whole range of other pigments.

So again, always go for a whole food source of phytochemicals, if you can. Researchers at Cleveland Clinic conducted a meta-analysis, combining the results of eight studies on the effects of beta-carotene at doses ranging from 15 to 50 milligrams. After investigating data from over 130,000 patients, researchers found that supplementation of beta carotene (most of that supplements to be truthful was synthetic form of carotene) led to a small increase in cardiovascular death (Use of antioxidant vitamins for the prevention of cardiovascular disease: meta-analysis of randomized trials. Lancet. 2003 Jun 14;361(9374):2017-23). Oil-soluble antioxidants like vitamin E and beta carotene are important for the prevention of heart disease because oxidized LDL is thought to play an important part in the pathogenesis of atherosclerosis. Observational studies have associated alpha-tocopherol (vitamin E), beta carotene, and other oil-soluble pigments and antioxidants with reductions in cardiovascular events but again this is from food sources of these antioxidants. When researched in the supplemental form it was a different story. Because beta carotene is an oil-soluble substance, the absorption will be increased if you add some nuts or seeds to your carrots but if you really want a supplemental form of beta carotene then chose a natural sourced supplement and don't overdo with the amounts. There are much better supplemental antioxidants that don't have any negative effects and are tens and hundreds of times more potent then beta carotene or supplemental vitamin E. But again, vitamin E is a vitamin and have a vital role in body functioning and you need to take adequate amount of it in food or if you don't have enough from diet then take a supplement. There is also a misconception that because retinol or animal-sourced vitamin A is the "real" vitamin A that somehow our body will not absorb and utilize enough beta carotene in the vegan diet to make vitamin A so that vegans need to supplement with vitamin A. This is not correct. It is just one more myth. It can be true if you are what I like to call junk vegan that eat French fries and drinks Coca Cola, but if you eat a normal whole food vegan diet it is not a case. If you want to supplement there are some potent supplemental antioxidants that don't have any negative side-effects.

In past times there was strong resistance and it persists to this day from regular medical institutions against any form of supplemental antioxidants. In the past, it was so fierce that the medical establishment did everything it can to discourage people from taking antioxidants. The main "reason" or story was that antioxidants are not important to anything except preventing scurvy or direct vitamin E deficiency. Anything more than that was quackery. For decades it was a scientific battle because if there is some treatment like mega-dosing on vitamin C or E or other antioxidants then who is going to make money from patented drugs, chemotherapy, surgeries and all of the rest of it. I already analyzed some of the histories behind the medical business but there is truth that even today with thousands of studies there is no recommendation of daily antioxidant consumption. Antioxidants and other phytochemicals are never and I want to emphasize this, never talked or discussed and even if you want to use for example megadose of some antioxidant to treat some disease the doctor will threaten you, don't want to give the treatment to you, and even directly confront you. There was one good example of this when men named Allan Smith basically come back from the dead. It was a big legal scandal and ended up in a news and in tv shows and discussions in Parliament. He was infected with the swine flu and his immune system collapsed. He was in a coma and was on life support unable to breathe by himself. Doctors demanded from his family that he should be taken off life support and that there is nothing else that they can do, and that he is basically already dead. The family refused. Because his family knows about the work of Luis Pauling and his institute they rejected and demanded from the medical staff that he was to be injected directly with a mega-dose of vitamin C. In animals for example when they contract the infection the production of vitamin C dramatically increases. It is hard for people to understand how can antioxidants have an effect on viruses but the answer is very simple. If you go down deep enough to the molecular scale, every virus or toxin or anything like oxygen or some other substance is the same. All of them are just electron scavengers. Oxygen, viruses, and toxins on the molecular level exert their action by stealing electrons from other molecules. That is it. It can be snake poison or bird flu it does not matter. On the molecular level, they are just seeking to take electrons from other molecules and vitamin C is a water-soluble antioxidant that has that one extra electron. The family of Allan Smith knowing all of this demanded that he is to be given megadose of intravenous vitamin C. And the medical doctors refused. They were so enraged by this that they told the family that they will not give any vitamin C and that they will turn off the machines without their consent. This is very psychological and existential for MD's because if there is a cure for such strong viruses like swine flu and that cure cannot be patented then their entire profession is obsolete and not just that, their entire profession is guilty of murdering millions of people by withholding therapies that they cannot charge for. Every time when you want to do this expect violence in every imaginable form. MD's are not nice, there are not here to heal you, and don't really care if you die as long as they can have six-figure salaries. Allan's lung was so filled with infected fluid that he was not able to take any air what so ever and in the eyes of MD's he was already dead with no chances what so ever of any recovery. They didn't "believe" in the quackery of Luis Pauling that was "proven" by the FDA that antioxidants and vitamin C are just there to prevent scurvy and the story was done. No discussion and you don't have a right to tell them what the truth is because who are you, some idiot that believes in pseudoscience. After three weeks in a coma, he was diagnosed with leukemia on top of that and specialists told the family that they will turn off the life support. This was all documented, 60 minutes

TV show managed to get hold of Auckland Hospital record from that meeting where they decided to turn off the life support and to this day Auckland Hospital remained silent about incident and never gave any public statement hoping that this story will eventually be forgotten. When they told his family that they are going to end his life the family demanded megadose of intravenous vitamin C. They said no. Then the family became angry telling the doctors that they don't have to believe anything there is nothing that they can lose if this doesn't work and that if they refuse to do this, they will call a lawyer. Then the Auckland board decided to wait two more days and they gave one injection on Thursday night of 25g vitamin C and then one more injection of 25 grams on Wednesday morning. Wednesday night they did a scan of his chest and they found air pockets. On x-ray just two days apart, the lung dramatically improved beyond anything that was naturally possible. The argument of the medical staff was that he got better because they turned him one day before that on a stomach. In reality, they were stricken by fear and they didn't know what to do now. They wanted to end his life, but now because he is showing dramatical improvement they could not. At the same time, this will prove that they were wrong in the first place. But again, they could not be wrong because then the entire medical industry is wrong or worse, a scam designed to kill people. So, they made up an excuse that vitamin C had nothing to do with this. Then the family asked them if turning him on a stomach had an impact on a such dramatical improvement why they did not try that before they decided to turn the machine off? There was no answer. After just 5 days of intravenous vitamin C, Allen improved to the point where he was able to breathe on his own and could be taken off the life support and on Friday he was taken off. But now his condition again started to deteriorate and was on a brink of going back to the life support again with fluids filling his lungs. The family found out that the medical board has put another consultant in and that new consultant has taken him off the vitamin C. The new consultant was so against it that he was not willing to administer any more vitamin C and didn't care about any posable lawsuit against him. He was just sitting in his chair and saying no, not going to do this, no, not putting him back on, no, you do whatever you want, no, not putting him back on. Then one of the Allen sons got "angry" and the meeting was stopped. Then the board put him back on, but only on 1 gram a day. The dose was very low but unfortunately to the medical board, he started to recover again, just at a slower rate. Then he was transferred to another hospital and again doctors there took him off from that low dose of vitamin C again. Then the family finally called a lawyer and filed a lawsuit against the hospital and decided to go to the high court of New Zeeland. Then the doctors put him back on but again, they administrated a low dose of 2 grams a day and the family wanted 50 grams a day. Eventually, a family discovered that you can megadose orally with vitamin C without any injection. When you take vitamin C in a powder form our body cannot absorb all of that vitamin C at once but there is a form of vitamin C that is captured in a lipid molecule to trick the body. It is called liposomal vitamin C and when the body absorbs that lipids and starts to break them down, vitamin C gets released. The family started to supplement him after he was out of the coma and the hospital was unable to stop them legally. He was awoken and he, by his own free will, can take any supplement he wants even without doctor's consent. He was told that it will take three months for him to be able to walk and after he woke and started to take liposomal vitamin C on his own, he was out of there in 14 days. Also, as a side note, his leukemia was healed also. This story became a political issue in New Zeeland and was on the news and the lesson here is, when you want intravenous vitamin C administered to you or a family member in the hospital, you don't tell your doctor. You instead tell your lawyer to tell your doctor in writing form. Lypo C is a good source of antioxidants because the body can use extra electrons from it to neutralize toxins and then can urinate out the oxidized form of vitamin C (dehydroascorbic acid). For our organism, it is easy to remove an oxidized form of vitamin C and other types of water-soluble antioxidants through our kidneys when they became pro-oxidants. This effectively keeps us in a surplus of free electrons. For example, in this study (Dehydroascorbic acid in urine as a possible indicator of surgical stress. Ann Nutr Metab. 2003;47(1):1-5) they concluded that surgery increases the oxidation of AA (ascorbic acid) and urinary excretion of DHAA (dehydroascorbic acid), as a result of the enhanced formation of free radicals. Any stress to the body, not just surgery will take some of that free electrons from excessive mega-dosed vitamin C to neutralize inflammation so at any time where there is a need for excessive antioxidant intake it is scientifically proven today, no matter what some MD is preaching, that mega dosing of vitamin C is beneficial. But when you are dealing with oil-soluble antioxidants like vitamin E and beta carotene then excessive amounts of them have to be removed through enzymatic pathways and it is much more complicated than just urinating it out. This can be a reason why you can take mega doses of vitamin C basically with no correlation to any disease or mortality unlike vitamin E for example where there is a point of diminishing returns. But again, most of the studies that exist use a synthetic form of vitamin E not natural form and I believe that this is done on purpose. Regular medicine does not like cheap and effective solutions that cannot be patented. When you mention antioxidants or in this case, vitamin C to the MD be prepare for a burst of hate. You are endangering their six-figure salaries and they don't like it one bit.

So far, science is conflicted but there is somewhat of a consensus. In normal circumstances in healthy individuals, the body will automatically maintain the level of vitamin C in the bloodstream. The RDA for vitamin C is set as same as for any other vitamin and that is the minimum level that is capable of preventing scurvy. Absolute minuscule amount when compared to the real optimal level. The regular medicine doesn't think of vitamin C in the same way that natural healers do. They think of vitamin C as a vitamin that has a role in preventing deficiency and diseases like scurvy but when we take vitamin C, we and actually our bodies use it as an antioxidant as well. Most people that supplement with vitamin C also supplement not because they have a need to prevent scurvy but to utilize the antioxidant power of that vitamin. When we think of vitamin C, we think of the antioxidant potential of ascorbic acid and the way we can use it to enhance our health and prevent a wide range of diseases. Scurvy has nothing to do with it. So, what might be the optimal intake of vitamin C? The easiest way to see the real need for this antioxidant is to measure the levels that our bodies absorb when we mega-dose with it and to measure the levels of excretion. If we take for example 15mg of vitamin C we will absorb 89 percent of it but if you take a supplement that has 1250mg of it the body will absorb 49 percent (Authors' perspective: What is the optimum intake of vitamin C in humans? doi: 10.1080/10408398.2011.649149). Up to the 200mg a day, our body will absorb all of it. A single orange has about 70mg of vitamin C. Then as we go up the absorption will decline. The overall absorption in mg will still go up but the percentage of absorption will decrease. In normal conditions, our body's evolved to absorb at least 200mg of it a day and maybe some percentage more than that. In addition, in our kidneys, vitamin C is reabsorbed back into the bloodstream to maintain our blood levels in the range of about 70 to 80 micromoles per liter and that is the level we can reach in vitamin C intake of about 200mg per day. In normal conditions even if we megadose with 5000mg the kidneys will excrete it to maintain the level of about 80 micromoles. So, the real RDA for vitamin C is 200mg in normal conditions and current acknowledged RDA by the medical establishment for adult nonsmoking men and women is 60 mg/d. But again, this is also partially the truth. You have seen me write more than once "in normal conditions". When we have abnormal exposure to toxins or infections of any sort the body will absorb as much as it can. When you are not sick and you take vitamin C in the oral form there will be a point when you will suffer from vitamin C induced diarrhea. If you have constipation this might help you as a natural cure. The level of this threshold for megadose induced vitamin C diarrhea is individual. This threshold is about 2000 to 3000mg for adult healthy male depending on your overall inflammation level and overall antioxidant intake. If you smoke and eat junk and your antioxidant intake is negligible your threshold will go up. People that have cancer or AIDS can take in some cases as much as 30 grams of it without having a laxative effect. There are thousands of cases, and this is well documented, and there is a line of research in recent years on the anticancer effect of vitamin C. In one case that I know a man had prostate cancer and simple do-it-yourself oral vitamin C protocol. It was recommended to him by an "underground" cancer treatment expert whose name I cannot use publicly. Initially, he reached bowel tolerance taking 60 grams per day. After two months his tolerance was down to less than 30 grams per day. But now we have something that will go against the interests of the drug industry and if you read the second part of the series you know what this means.

Actually, it all started with one man, Linus Pauling. He was named as a quack, renegade, delusional scientist and all other "names" you can think of. It was a standard strategy of propaganda and slander of Big Pharma cartels. But in this case, there was a problem also. Linus Carl Pauling (1901-1994) was a physical chemist and father of biochemistry who won two Nobel Prize awards; one in chemistry in 1954, followed by a Nobel Peace Prize in 1962. He should have won the third Nobel as well but powers at be decided that that was not good for the business and gave it to Watson and Crick for "narrowly" beating him to the discovery of the structure of DNA. The New Scientist magazine ranked him as one of the 20 greatest scientists to ever live. At one time he did research into vitamin C and understood the biochemistry behind the antioxidants and their ability to neutralize the toxic substances, free radicals and to kill off viruses. He wrote a book on the subject of vitamin C where he advocated mega-dosing to utilize vitamin C antioxidant potential to prevent the cold and because of his reputation the book was a bestseller. Sales of vitamin C soared with Pauling endorsement. But he was naive. He was convinced that he had discovered a new cure for many illnesses and that medical professionals will be happy because they can heal people with something that is cheap and don't need prescription and that MD's won't be wasting time anymore on people with common cold for which they didn't have any treatment at that time anyway. But he was wrong. Attacks were launched immediately. First from Harvard and professor Frederic Stair calling him an idiot that doesn't know anything about nutrition and that he is not a physician but just a chemist and that he doesn't know anything about what he is talking about in the area of nutrition. Pauling's recommendation was a minimum of 6 grams per day and he was extrapolating at that time the amounts of vitamin C that was prescribed by a veterinary medicine for the primates in the zoos. He calculated the RDA for primates with their body weight and just recalculated and recommended the same amount to humans. It was heresy. That was 200 times what was officially recommended. The real problem was the fear that this might actually work and that the medical professionals will be left without a big chunk of the prescription drugs income. Pauling was arguing that vitamin C as an antioxidant has a value of boosting body natural defense mechanisms and can heal not just common cold but a range of other diseases such as cancer and many others as well, and not just that. He argued that mega dosing will increase longevity and quality of life. In allopathic (modern) medicine, if you have a "magical" cure that heals every disease and gives you the longevity you are a quack. If you have two Nobel's and are the "father" of the biochemistry, and you have such a substance that is also dirt cheap you are not just a quack, you are a threat. Pauling next step hit the medical establishment right to the sacrosanct area of making money. He wrote a book based on medical records of patients that have been treated with high doses of vitamin C by the Scottish surgeon dr. Ewen Cameron. Both Cameron and Pauling claimed that antioxidants like vitamin C can stop the damage of DNA and prevent cancer and if patients already have one that vitamin C can prolong life with no side effects of chemotherapy. In 1966, Cameron published his first book, Hyaluronidase and Cancer. In 1971, Cameron began corresponding with Dr. Linus Pauling and published Cancer and Vitamin C with Pauling in 1979. Pauling still not realizing the scope of corruption, took the data from his research and went to American National Cancer Institute. The response was that he is a quack and danger to society and that he needs to stop his heresy and that they are not going to do any research. Because they couldn't silence him or make him go away, and because of the public awareness, the pressure was mounting and the Mayo Clinic decided to do a research. The Mayo Clinic study was stopped after 75 days and was giving low doses of oral not intravenous vitamin C and was designed in a way that Pauling consider as a fraud. He wrote a serious of letters to the medical journals claiming it to be a conspiracy. He was rebuffed and called a dangerous quack and actually both his own wife and dr. Cameron, both died from cancer. Pauling even after that didn't give up his theory and still was promoting his antioxidant theory and had his own laboratory where he did research that exists to this day. It is Linus Pauling Institute near San Francisco that has around 40 scientific staff and to this day is financed by private benefactors inspired by the cause. They tested vitamin C on cholesterol and heart disease and published a series of papers on lowering the effects of vitamin C on cholesterol and more importantly on oxidation of cholesterol. The medical branch just rejects all of his studies and that is that.

At the end who was right, was it all a conspiracy? The answer is yes, it was all a conspiracy to protect the model of business. Forty years later we now know exactly what oxidation does to the DNA and we know exactly what antioxidants and in this case vitamin C does. For example here is a study from 2015 from Singapore (Effects of High Doses of Vitamin C on Cancer Patients in Singapore doi: 10.1177/1534735415622010) with a conclusion: "Compared with chemotherapy, IVC therapy, in combination with a diet and supplement regimen, is tolerated well, appears to have antitumor activity in some cases, has been administered alongside conventional therapy without impairing response, is safe for most patients, and is inexpensive. It also appears to increase the quality of life for patients. IVC therapy has the potential to become an important chemotherapeutic method to combat cancer. This, however, can take place only through further research and clinical study." So where are American National Cancer Institute and Mayo Clinic now to give these scientists the titles like quacks and senile megalomaniacs? Here are some quotes from the study: "After IVC (intravenous vitamin C) treatment, P2 showed necrotic activity in his abnormal enlarged cervical lymph nodules that had not been removed by the previous radiotherapy. The invasive breast carcinoma in P7 disappeared after 6 months. Most remarkably, the tumor P8 had been afflicted with shrank by 49.3% in the first 21 days of intensive IVC therapy. This was followed by a 93% shrinkage after approximately 6 weeks. The patient was totally cleared 10 months later. P9 also showed remarkable tumor shrinkage. After the relapse of cancer in 2009, the patient did not seek conventional treatment and decided to solely focus on IVC therapy. For P9, his tumor also shrank from $11.3 \times 10.7 \times 7.5$ to $7.1 \times 6.6 \times 6.0$ cm3 for the whole duration of IVC therapy. On the other hand, when P5 stopped IVC therapy, her breast tumor growth started to worsen. Her tumor grew from $6 \times 5.6 \times 4.2$ to $6.6 \times 6 \times 3.7$ cm3 in a span of less than 5 months. When P5 initially started IVC therapy, her 3 tumors showed consistent results: shrinkage of 30% to 53%. These improvements in her tumor were seen in a span of 1 month. P5's tumor growth only started to worsen after the removal of IVC therapy and illustrated the likelihood of tumor regression attributed to IVC therapy."

This study is just one example, by now there are thousands of studies done on mega-dosing vitamin C but guess what, nobody will ever tell the patients this. Vitamin C is cheap, vitamin C cannot be patented and vitamin C is effective. And keep in mind that vitamin C is not, in reality, a very strong antioxidant. It is actually weak compared to some other available antioxidants but when you take a huge amount of it and inject it directly to the vain then you can compensate for its weak strength by giving a higher dose of it. And the body has the ability to urinate out the oxidized form of vitamin C because it is the water-soluble antioxidant with no problem and with no use of any enzymes in the process. The end effect will be the absorption of free electrons and neutralization of oxidative and other toxic agents inside the body. Everything that vitamin C was able to do, it was able to do because of its antioxidative properties. There is nothing unique that vitamin C has that other antioxidants do not have. They are all on a molecular level just electron donors, and that is it. Luis Pauling was right. He was ostracized and he was willing to take that risk and didn't care about what corrupted clinics as Mayo do. He personally wanted his heresy to be his legacy not the title of father of biochemistry and molecular biology or Nobel prizes. He wanted to be remembered as a vitamin C man that brought to light the importance of antioxidants and revolution in human medicine. Antioxidants do prevent DNA from damage and do prolong life and if you have less inflammation you will have less mutation and fewer cancer cells living inside you and you will have an immune system that is not overloaded with toxins that can actually kill off all of the cancer cells before they became the problem and not just that. Antioxidants and in particular vitamin C directly kill the cancer cells as well. Dr. Riordan carried out a 15-year long research project called RECNAC (cancer spelled backward). His research in cell cultures showed that vitamin C was selectively cytotoxic against cancer cells. The mechanism for this is summarized by Dr. Hunninghake:

"Cancer cells were actively taking up vitamin C in a way that depleted tissue reserves. PET scans are commonly ordered by oncologists to evaluate their cancer patients for metastases (cancer spread to other organs).

What is actually injected into the patient at the start of the scan is radioactive glucose. Cancer cells... depend upon glucose as their primary source of metabolic fuel... [and] employ transport mechanisms called glucose transporters to actively pull in glucose.

In the vast majority of animals, vitamin C is synthesized from glucose in only four metabolic steps. Hence, the molecular shape of vitamin C is remarkably similar to glucose. Cancer cells will actively transport vitamin C into themselves, possibly because they mistake it for glucose. Another plausible explanation is that they are using vitamin C as an antioxidant. Regardless, vitamin C accumulates in cancer cells.

If large amounts of vitamin C are presented to cancer cells, large amounts will be absorbed. In these unusually large concentrations, the antioxidant vitamin C will start behaving as a pro-oxidant as it interacts with intracellular copper and iron. This chemical interaction produces small amounts of hydrogen peroxide.

Because cancer cells are relatively low in an intracellular anti-oxidant enzyme called catalase, the high dose vitamin C induction of peroxide will continue to build up until it eventually lyses the cancer cell from the inside out! This effectively makes high dose IVC a non-toxic chemotherapeutic agent that can be given in conjunction with conventional cancer treatments. "

You don't have to megadose on vitamin C because the body does not have the ability to store it. It is a water-soluble antioxidant. If you take vitamin C on a regular base you will have some of the benefits but still, most of it will be excreted out with the urine. The best approach is to eat antioxidant-rich whole foods and if you like you can take supplements and some of them are much more superior then vitamin C. Technology had come a long way since the 1970s and I will describe some of the supplements that I recommend later. If you have the swine flu or cancer then intravenous vitamin C is the must. If you have cancer you never have to get off of it. Unlike chemotherapy, there are no vitamin C side effects. It is chemotherapy that can be taken for the rest of your life and just this fact is what terrifies the regular cancer industry. The intravenous vitamin C shots are expensive and so is the liposomal vitamin C. There are videos on YouTube where people are trying to make their own liposomal vitamin C at home with just lecithin and ascorbic acid mixed in together then energized inside ultrasonic cleaner for encapsulation. Does this work, I don't really know. Liposomal encapsulation is a process where fat is used to encapsulate some molecules inside it. In this case, it is vitamin C so when cells metabolize the fat the inner part of the compound gets released. It is a nice way to trick the body. Liposomal vitamin C also gets released inside the cell not into the bloodstream so it is more potent even then intravenous vitamin C because not all of the ascorbic acid that is in the blood will get absorbed into the cells. When ascorbic acid is in the blood there are molecules known as transporters that take that vitamin C and integrate it into the cell but when phosphatidylcholine encapsulated vitamin C comes into contact with a cell there is no need for transport because cells pass through phospholipids right in. Phosphatidylcholine is a fat molecule that cell membranes are made of. When ascorbic acid is in the blood then some will be urinated out. In liposomal encapsulation, all of the vitamin C goes directly to the cells inside the body. If you want to make homemade liposomal vitamin C you need to understand that phospholipids are not the same as lecithin. They are extracted from lecithin and commercial products are the real deal, however, I don't know if homemade liposomals have any effectiveness at all or are they as potent as pharma grade. Doctors that do vitamin C as a treatment generally consider 1000mg of liposomal vitamin C to be as effective as 15000mg of oral vitamin C and liposomal form does not cause a laxative effect. If we really go into it, we can see that mega-dosing on universal antioxidants and antioxidants that do not have enzymatic breakdown metabolism like in this case liposomal vitamin C have the ability to easily wipe out more than 50 percent of prescription medications, from different types of chemotherapy onward. And the medical industry will do everything and I will say this again, the medical industry will do anything to forbid you to use it. You will literary have to call a lawyer to force the MD to give you an intravenous ascorbic acid. And it is not a coincidence or misinformation but as Pauling use to say, it is a well-organized conspiracy. Mega-dosing of liposomal ascorbic acid encapsulation is also good for an overall state of inflammation but especially for inflamed gums and teeth. Vitamin C stimulates the immune system by more than 20 identified mechanisms. Low level of painless inflammation is something that most people don't realize that they have because of the toxic overload and bad diet but in the long run, it will kill you. Taking liposomal vitamin C, plus eating high quality antioxidant-rich whole plant food diet will have a big impact on the immune system, overall lowering of inflammation, prevention of cancer, prevention of periodontal diseases, prevention of infections from different viruses and overall longevity and well-being. Eating animal products that do not have any type of antioxidant in them but just a high level of dead meat bacteria will create endotoxemia and inflammation. Plus if we add on top of that a whole range of pollutants from the environment it is a recipe for chronic, in initial stages painless inflammation, then a whole range of painful diseases in stage two like cancer and then shortening of lifespan and death. There is also evidence that vitamin C can lower the cortisol level and could mitigate stress response in rats, both in terms of regular stress or sleep deprivation (Vitamin C Prevents Sleep Deprivation-induced Elevation in Cortisol and Lipid Peroxidation in the Rat Plasma Niger. J. Physiol. Sci. 30(2015) 005-009) or exercise (Vitamin C supplementation attenuates the increases in circulating cortisol, adrenaline and anti-inflammatory polypeptides following ultramarathon running. Int J Sports Med. 2001 Oct;22(7):537-43). At least in the case of plasma cortisol, which could help to improve stress tolerance. Elevated cortisol levels can induce a state of insomnia and fatigue and anxiety. Cortisol is a hormone released by the adrenal glands in response to stress. If you drink coffee and on top of that have a bad diet that creates inflammation the response of the body will be to increase cortisol levels to fight that inflammation. It is the strongest anti-inflammatory hormone in the body. Corticosteroids are prescribed for inflammation as well. But besides lowering inflammation once it gets into the bloodstream, cortisol is also responsible for relaying the news of stress to all parts of the body and mind. Cortisol is the hormone that triggers the so-called "fight or flight" response to stress. Evolutionary is a hormone that puts the body and mind in a survival state. It is an essential hormone to life. But if we are overexposed to stress, high levels of stress hormones will exhaust the body's physical resources, impair learning and memory, and will make people susceptible to depression. If you have issues with anxiety and adrenal insufficiency vitamin C can help. It helps to reduce both the physical and psychological effects of stress on people. One more plant that has phytochemicals that are known to have a lowering of cortisol and epinephrine effects is Rooibos (Aspalathus linearis) that is commonly consumed as tea (Rooibos Flavonoids Inhibit the Activity of Key Adrenal Steroidogenic Enzymes, Modulating Steroid Hormone Levels in H295R Cells doi: 10.3390/molecules19033681). Flavones from the tea have an effect of binding and neutralizing enzymes that adrenal glands use to make glucocorticoid hormones like cortisol and epinephrine. These flavones decreased levels of cortisol and epinephrine by 4 times. Researches were alarmed that they might even lower testosterone levels but it was not the case. Rooibos tea just lowered the circulating glucocorticoid levels. And it is a natural way of lowering stress response in the form of a cup or two of tea in a day. When looking at vitamin C the extrapolated doses for people stress management will be around 1,000 mg. It is a dose that was found to be helpful in the stress study. If you want to increase vitamin C intake naturally by the food intake you need to know that vitamin C is destroyed by cooking and exposure to light. If you want to take a supplement and don't want liposomal form then the best way is to take it is in a time-released preparation that works over the course of a day. Another solution would be to take vitamin C supplements in time intervals throughout the day.

If we compare vitamin C to other phytochemicals that have antioxidative properties we will see that vitamin C is actually pretty week antioxidant. Some of the plant pigments are very strong and much stronger than vitamin C. These pigments sole purpose is to defend the plant from solar radiation and oxidation. The reason why we have color vision unlike carnivores is exactly this, so that we can identify these plant pigments, so that we can eat them because our body needs this protection as well and so that we can identify ripe fruits because of the energy stored in them in form of fructose. Millions of years of evolution that gave us color vision is a much more important recommendation than a recommendation from the medical establishment. These plant pigments are essential to us as much as any other vitamin with only one difference. We will not die from antioxidant deficiency directly. We will die indirectly from cancer or some other chronic disease and we will have an increase in cellular aging and inflammation and a shorter life. The stronger the pigment the stronger is his power for neutralizing free radicals. Some of the plants that have strong pigments are the healthiest and have the most positive effects on our bodies. For example, berries are universally accepted as the healthiest fruit because of their strong antioxidative properties. Berries have very strong pigments. For instance, acai berries are so strong that they are used for staining people digestive tract before imaging with x-rays. Some other plants have even stronger pigments than berries like turmeric. It will stain everything it touches. Small pinch of turmeric is enough to make your entire dish yellow. It is one of the strongest pigments out there. Curcumin is actually so health-promoting and so protective that it is researched as a chemotherapy drug besides a wide range of other implications. Elemene, for example, is phytochemical derived from turmeric and is approved in China for the treatment of cancer. Curcumin is the main yellow pigment in turmeric that was found to have the most protective properties. We have to keep in mind that curcumin is just one of the many phytochemicals in turmeric. There is a whole list of other active ingredients in turmeric as a whole plant but the reductionist mentality of the medical industry believes that it is much more effective and of course, much more lucrative practice if the active ingredient is extracted and then mega dosed in a pill form.

Plants contain numerous polyphenols, which have been shown to reduce inflammation and thereby will increase resistance to disease. Examples of such polyphenols are isothiocyanates in cabbage and broccoli, epigallocatechin in green tee, capsaicin in chili peppers, chalones, rutin and naringenin in apples, resveratrol in red wine and fresh peanuts. But it is impossible to research them all. Only in turmeric there are more than 300 active phytochemicals so far identified. For example, in this study (Curcumin-free turmeric exhibits anti-inflammatory and anticancer activities: Identification of novel components of turmeric. doi: 10.1002/mnfr.201200838) they concluded that turmeric deprived of curcumin is more effective in fighting cancer and has more anti-inflammatory effects than curcumin by itself. The problem is that turmeric is just a spice and it is dirt cheap so no patents at the end of the research if not extracted to some pill form. The conclusion of the study was that turmeric represents a good source of new chemicals for the medical industry, not that people should eat the whole turmeric as a medicinal herb.

There is a problem with curcumin and that is his poor bioavailability. When consumed only tiny amounts will end up being utilized. Supplements use different methods to increase the bioavailability to up to 99 percent. They are more convenient to take but the whole food source is much healthier because of the wide range of different phytochemicals in it. Ideally, the solution would be to take the spice as whole food produce and to increase its absorption. There is a way that we can do that. The solution is black pepper. There is a phytochemical in black pepper that boosts the bioavailability of curcumin if consumed together. Curcumin is approximately 5% of the weight of turmeric. Also, about 5% of black pepper by weight is comprised of phytochemical called piperine. Piperine is what gives black pepper its aroma but it is also a strong inhibitor of liver metabolism. There are different pathways that the liver uses to detoxify chemicals and one of them is to make oil chemicals to be water-soluble so that they can be removed by kidneys. Piperine molecule inhibits that process and doesn't allow the liver to get rid of curcumin. When we add just a pinch of black pepper to turmeric 1/20th of a teaspoon the bioavailability of curcumin shoots up 2000% (Influence of piperine on the pharmacokinetics of curcumin in animals and human volunteers. Planta Med. 1998 May;64(4):353-6). Also, the same way as with any other pigment like for example beta carotene or lycopene (red pigment) from tomatoes the bioavailability of these compounds is greatly increased by adding oil to the meal. Fat can enhance the bioavailability of curcumin seven to eightfold. When eaten with fat, curcumin can be directly absorbed into the bloodstream through the lymphatic system thereby in part bypassing the liver. Adding a small amount of fat to the salads was found to have the same effect of a wide range of different oil-soluble phytochemicals. Actually, all oil-soluble phytochemicals and this includes the pigments will have higher absorption with oil and higher bioavailability with black pepper. The only real problem is high levels of bioavailable oxalates in turmeric. Oxalates can bind to calcium to form an insoluble calcium oxalate, which is responsible for approximately 75% of all kidney stones. In people who have tendencies to form kidney stones, the consumption of oxalates should be less than 40 to 50 mg/day, which means no more than at most a teaspoon of turmeric. People with kidney stones or gout that want to use turmeric to lower inflammation might consider using curcumin supplements because to reach high levels of curcumin from turmeric would incur too much of an oxalate load. One more thing that we have to take into account when dealing with turmeric is that it might trigger gallbladder pain in individuals with gallstones. It is a strong so-called cholecystokinetic agent, meaning that it facilitates the pumping action of the gallbladder to keep the bile from stagnating so if you have a stone in there the squeezing could cause a pain. So far in the last decade or so there was extensive research in turmeric and curcumin. Turmeric has been proven to dramatically lower inflammation for example in smokers and also helps in autoimmune inflammatory diseases from inflammatory bowel disease to osteoarthritis and rheumatoid arthritis, ulcerative colitis. It directly kills different types of cancer cells from colon, prostate, breast to pancreas like any other chemotherapy drug. It is very potent and at the same time, it does not have any negative side effects. It helps with diabetes type 2 and prediabetes and obesity and has strong neuroprotective properties. It helps with Alzheimer's disease, Parkinson's disease, regular cognitive decline, and even depression. It is good for arterial function. It can help with heavy metal exposure and other toxins. Everything ever tested basically gave a positive result and the truth is that actually there is nothing special about turmeric at all. It is just one more natural pigment or antioxidant like any other pigment. It is just stronger than some other pigments and that is it. But what is important to understand is that all pigments act similarly in the plants and in the human body. All pigments have protective properties, not just curcumin. Keep in mind that studies on the biochemistry of one pigment would be similar to all pigments that exist. It is the same principle. Some pigments and antioxidants will be stronger, some weaker, but on the molecular level, they all act the same by giving off an extra electron. For example, in cancer research in more scientific terms curcumin is known to modulate the activation of various transcription factors, it regulates the expression of inflammatory enzymes, cytokines, adhesion molecules, and cell survival proteins. In studies, it has proven to be an antiproliferative, anti-invasive, and antiangiogenic, as a mediator of chemoresistance, chemopreventive, and as a therapeutic agent (Research on curcumin: A meta-analysis of potentially malignant disorders. doi: 10.4103/0973-1482.171370). It modulates multiple molecular pathways involved in the carcinogenesis process: scavenging reactive oxidative species (ROS), reducing the inflammatory cancer microenvironment, promoting apoptosis (cell death) and by inhibiting survival signals (New perspectives of curcumin in cancer prevention. doi: 10.1158/1940-6207.CAPR-12-0410). There are hundreds of different genes that need to be mutated to create a cancer cell. Some estimates are between 300 and 500. Usually, most types of cancer start to develop in the teenage years and even before that but it takes decades until they are fully diagnosed and visible. That is because there are multiple different pathways that create different mutations that at the end will result in the formation of a malignant cancer cell. The problem is that when the medical industry deals with cancer and creates different chemotherapy drugs that drugs target only one pathway and are extremely specific in what they do. There is no holistic approach in the treatment of cancer and as a result, there is no drug regimen that will target all of those different pathways of cancer promotion. Plants phytochemicals and in this case curcumin does exactly that. That is the reason why in the last decade and especially since 2004 there is an explosion in turmeric research. Drug companies want to extract some of the phytochemicals from different plants that are known to have anti-cancer properties to use them in addition to already existing and narrow targeted chemotherapy drugs regiments to have more of multitargeted therapies, especially because the current practice has become unsustainable. People are educating themselves and starting to ask questions and starting to use the internet for their own research. Almost 50 years after President Richard Nixon signed the bill pushed by Big Pharma that would be called War on Cancer, cancer is still right behind heart disease as the leading cause of death in the United States. The numbers that they don't want you to know are something like this. When we look at real data of survival that all of the radiation and chemotherapy brings to someone life it is about 2.1 percent in the US (The contribution of cytotoxic chemotherapy to 5-year survival in adult malignancies. Clin Oncol (R Coll Radiol). 2004 Dec;16(8):549-60). I want to repeat this again. It is at 2.1 percent. Basically, all of that suffering is for nothing. Five years after the chemo the number of people that will still be alive compared to ones that did not receive any treatment is 2.1 percent. Actually, the real number is around 1 percent for most common cancers like colon, lung, breast and for prostate is zero. The average goes up one percent because there are some cancers like testicular or Hodgins that have survival rate much higher, about 40 percent but for more than 95% of different cancer types, it is basically zero. I wrote more about the Big Pharma medical business in the second part of the book series. This is not by accident or because the science is not adequate and cannot do anything about cancer. Around 95% of all cancers are caused by a bad diet and environmental toxicity plus all of the bad habits that increase our toxic overload like smoking and around 10 to 15 percent are caused by bad genes (Cancer is a preventable disease that requires major lifestyle changes. doi: 10.1007/s11095-008-9661-9). This is not a big secret except "they" just don't want to tell patients all of this. Cancer is 95 percent preventable disease, the same way as cardiovascular disease is or all of the other diseases of affluence that I already wrote about in the first book of the series.

Today big companies have started to invest in research into these phytochemicals more than they are been willing in the past with the desire to patent some of the phytochemicals as an end result and rise survival rate a little bit. But who can stop us from just eating them in a whole food manner? If we look at the statistics, we will see that population data shows that in India for example where turmeric is consumed in a significant amount there is a big gap in cancer rates then in western countries. In the U.S. the skin cancer rate with all of the sunscreen promotion from the dermatologists is 14 times more prominent than in India. That is 1400 percent more. Prostate cancer is 23 times more prominent, colorectal cancer 11 times more, endometrial cancer is 9 times, breast cancer 5 times, lung cancer 17 times and so on (Plant-derived health: the effects of turmeric and curcuminoids. Nutr Hosp. 2009 May-Jun;24(3):273-81). This is not just because of the turmeric but because of the fact that more than 40 percent of India's population is vegetarian and that people that do eat meat also eat much less of it on a daily bases than in the USA. On top of this, they consume much more vegetables and especially fruit and on top of this, they consume turmeric and other spices much more. The cancer rate difference in some types of cancers is even more prominent than the ones that are found in the China Study, but the conclusion is the same. How much does a high consumption rate of turmeric plays a role is an object of investigation, and you can read more on the topic if you want in this review (Dietary turmeric potentially reduces the risk of cancer. Asian Pac J Cancer Prev. 2011;12(12):3169-73). Currently, there is a lot of research done and turmeric is tested for a wide variety of cancers if not for all of them for both prevention and as a chemotherapy drug. Prevention is the keyword here. Phytochemicals do not have any negative side effects and do a lot of other beneficial things for other diseases and longevity and can be taken for extended periods of time or for our entire life and are cheap. Chemotherapy not so much and this is a crucial difference. It was known back in the 80s after some in vitro studies that curcumin blocks all three stages of cancer development cancer transformation, proliferation, and invasion. It even blocks mutagens to enter the cells in the first place so it has strong antitoxic and antimutagenic action. It also upregulates a lot of different pathways for apoptosis (self-induced cell death) in cancer cells but leaves normal cells alone with a mechanism not so fully understood. It will activate the cell self-destruction gene in cancer cells by a wide range of different pathways. Cancer cells normally have this mechanism turned off completely and actually never die. In scientific terms: "Curcumin modulates growth of tumor cells through regulation of multiple cell signaling pathways including cell proliferation pathway (cyclin D1, c-myc), cell survival pathway (Bcl-2, Bcl-xL, cFLIP, XIAP, c-IAP1), caspase activation pathway (caspase-8, 3, 9), tumor suppressor pathway (p53, p21) death receptor pathway (DR4, DR5), mitochondrial pathways, and protein kinase pathway (JNK, Akt, and AMPK)." (Curcumin and cancer cells: how many ways can curry kill tumor cells selectively? doi: 10.1208/s12248-009-9128-x). This is all nice on a paper but what is real practical efficiency of curcumin in human testing? How strong is it? It depends on the type of cancer and the research is still going on. But in some cases, it is even stronger than leading chemotherapy drugs. For example, when it was tested for pancreatic cancer that is one of the worst types with a survival rate of zero it managed to kill some of the cancer cells in around 10 percent of subjects and in one subject cancer regressed 73 percent. The problem with any drug that is designed to kill cancer cells is that there are different mutations in them so if only 1 percent of cancer cells survive and are resilient that 1 percent will then continue to multiply and in time it will grow and be the same size as before. That is why prevention is the key. If you already have cancer it is highly unlikely that curcumin will save your life. The only hope is that cancer is localized and that it can be surgically removed. Once it has spread throughout the body survival rate is minimal. The good thing about curcumin is that it does not have any negative side effects and that no matter how bad your diet is, it can still help. In one study (Effect of turmeric on urinary mutagens in smokers. Mutagenesis. 1992 Mar;7(2):107-9) they measured how much mutagens are in the urine of the smokers by dripping it to bacteria culture and then measuring the damage to DNA. Adding turmeric in doses of just 1.5 g/day for 30 days lowered the urinary mutagens by more than 50 percent. The conclusion was: "These results indicate that dietary turmeric is an effective anti-mutagen and it may be useful in chemoprevention." In my opinion, this phytochemical is well researched and turmeric should be added as a medicinal herb for the duration of a whole life.

Besides cancer prevention one of the strongest effects of turmeric is lowering overall inflammation in the body. This can slow down the oxidation and DNA damage giving us longevity but can also help with inflammatory and autoimmune diseases. The problem with autoimmune diseases is that there is no cure when the immune system malfunctions and starts to attack our own cells. The only treatment is to take immune suppressive medication that has severe side effects ranging from leukemia and cancer to infertility. Turmeric and other antioxidants can help without any side effects. Lupus is one of the autoimmune diseases that attack the nucleus of the cell itself so it can attack any organ and is very hard to treat. People with a disease like lupus have their life turned into a nightmare. In this study (Oral supplementation of turmeric decreases proteinuria, hematuria, and systolic blood pressure in patients suffering from relapsing or refractory lupus nephritis: a randomized and placebo-controlled study. doi: 10.1053/j.jrn.2011.03.002) they gave turmeric to subjects with refractory (untreatable) lupus. After treatment, all subjects except one man, almost 99 percent of them got better and got better significantly. Side effects free. It is highly unlikely that turmeric will be prescribed as a treatment by your doctor if you have lupus but you can take it yourself and if it helps you can lower your medication. If you don't have lupus take it as well as an antioxidant-rich medical herb. When dealing with other harsh inflammatory diseases like for example inflamed bowel disease (Crohn's disease) first study ever done was done in 2005 by individual doctors themselves that decided to go against the medical industry and do study themselves with no financial backup. It took almost 50 years after the first discovery that curcumin had anti-inflammatory properties for some rogue doctors in New York to do a study (Curcumin therapy in inflammatory bowel disease: a pilot study Dig Dis Sci. 2005 Nov;50(11):2191-3). Four out of five subjects treated improved. Ulcerative Colitis is actually not that uncommon. Many people have inflamed intestines from more milder forms to severe forms. Treatment is ineffective and has harsh side effects that can cause inflammation through the body like inflamed liver, kidneys and pancreas plus pain, fever, vomiting and in 30 percent of cases full-blown infertility. After the completion of that study, other studies were done. Next year in Japan there was a full double-blind, placebo-controlled, large scale study (Curcumin maintenance therapy for ulcerative colitis: randomized, multicenter, double-blind, placebo-controlled trial. DOI: 10.1016/j.cgh.2006.08.008). They used only 2 grams of curcumin per day and actually admitted themselves that the dose is inadequate. Nevertheless, the result was a 5% relapse rate in the curcumin group compared to a 20% relapse rate in the control group. People that have Crohn's disease have autoimmune flare-ups or relapses but besides that, the overall state of curcumin group was much better both subjectively and objectively with the endoscopic examination. The difference was so extreme that researches could not believe the results and were theorizing that it might just be that for example people selected randomly were in better condition and are healthier just by some fluke coincidence. So, they decided to prolong the study for six more months but they gave everyone a placebo. They wanted to see would those people that were getting curcumin start to relapse once again after they have been taken off of it. That was exactly what happened and remember this was only 2 grams a day. Curcumin is a powerful substance. It is so powerful that it can even alter our gene expression. We are born with a fixed genetic structure but our genes constantly mutate and evolution goes forward. What genes would be activated depends on their expression that is dependent on environmental (external) factors.

The summary of this review (Molecular mechanisms of curcumin action: gene expression. doi: 10.1002/biof.1041) says it all: "The preventive and therapeutic properties of curcumin are associated with its antioxidant, anti-inflammatory, and anticancer properties. Extensive research over several decades has attempted to identify the molecular mechanisms of curcumin action. Curcumin modulates numerous molecular targets by altering their gene expression, signaling pathways, or through direct interaction. Curcumin regulates the expression of inflammatory cytokines (e.g., TNF, IL-1), growth factors (e.g., VEGF, EGF, FGF), growth factor receptors (e.g., EGFR, HER-2, AR), enzymes (e.g., COX-2, LOX, MMP9, MAPK, mTOR, Akt), adhesion molecules (e.g., ELAM-1, ICAM-1, VCAM-1), apoptosis related proteins (e.g., Bcl-2, caspases, DR, Fas), and cell cycle proteins (e.g., cyclin D1). Curcumin modulates the activity of several transcription factors (e.g., NF-$\varkappa$B, AP-1, STAT) and their signaling pathways. Based on its ability to affect multiple targets, curcumin has the potential for the prevention and treatment of various diseases including cancers, arthritis, allergies, atherosclerosis, aging, neurodegenerative disease, hepatic disorders, obesity, diabetes, psoriasis, and autoimmune diseases."

They have described aging in the review as a disease as well. I found that to be interesting, and yes strong antioxidants have the potential to protect DNA from damage and in a sense prolong life. You won't be able to understand any of this scientific terminology but that is not important. What is important is to understand the extent of the potency of certain medicinal plants and their phytochemicals. People tend to think that only synthetic molecules that come from some laboratory have any medical potential and the truth is completely opposite. The real potential is in phytochemicals that have been evolving for hundreds of millions of years on this planet and synthetic molecules are just weak substances that have been created so that big chemical companies can make a lot of money on their patents. And even most of the drugs today are actually just extracted phytochemicals in the first place. I will use a quote from a review that was done back in 2013, and this is from clinical trials on humans (Therapeutic roles of curcumin: lessons learned from clinical trials. doi: 10.1208/s12248-012-9432-8). They concluded: "Some promising effects have been observed in patients with various pro-inflammatory diseases including cancer, cardiovascular disease, arthritis, uveitis, ulcerative proctitis, Crohn's disease, ulcerative colitis, irritable bowel disease, tropical pancreatitis, peptic ulcer, gastric ulcer, idiopathic orbital inflammatory pseudotumor, oral lichen planus, gastric inflammation, vitiligo, psoriasis, acute coronary syndrome, atherosclerosis, diabetes, diabetic nephropathy, diabetic microangiopathy, lupus nephritis, renal conditions, acquired immunodeficiency syndrome, β-thalassemia, biliary dyskinesia, Dejerine-Sottas disease, cholecystitis, and chronic bacterial prostatitis. Curcumin has also shown protection against hepatic conditions, chronic arsenic exposure, and alcohol intoxication. Dose-escalating studies have indicated the safety of curcumin at doses as high as 12 g/day over 3 months. Curcumin's pleiotropic activities emanate from its ability to modulate numerous signaling molecules such as pro-inflammatory cytokines, apoptotic proteins, NF-$\varkappa$B, cyclooxygenase-2, 5-LOX, STAT3, C-reactive protein, prostaglandin E(2), prostate-specific antigen, adhesion molecules, phosphorylase kinase, transforming growth factor-β, triglyceride, ET-1, creatinine, HO-1, AST, and ALT in human participants."

On the other hand eating animal products have complete opposite action. Meat is not just a neutral product that is rich in iron and protein. It is a food item that is loaded with dead meat bacteria endotoxins and mutagens especially when cooked and has other toxins and heavy metals from environment and cholesterol and saturated fat and it stimulates cancer-promoting IGF-1 and is pro-inflammatory just by itself even if we disregard the fact that it does not have any of the antioxidant properties in a first place.

If you are young and completely healthy and if you have the healthiest diet that you possibly can you still should add curcumin and some other medicinal plants and supplements that have been shown to have health-promoting abilities. If not for anything else then just as a means of prolonging your life expectancy and protecting yourself from diseases in the long run. Turmeric also has strong neuroprotective properties that will help with neurological disorders and diseases but also with normal cognitive decline that goes with aging. It will help with prediabetes and obesity. It will help with artery function. In many of the inflammatory diseases it works better than leading drugs with no side effects. For example, 500 mg of curcumin works significantly better for rheumatoid arthritis than diclofenac (A randomized, pilot study to assess the efficacy and safety of curcumin in patients with active rheumatoid arthritis. doi: 10.1002/ptr.4639). Keep in mind that diclofenac is a very strong nonsteroidal anti-inflammatory drug that is also used for migraine attacks or kidney stones and other painful conditions and would also dramatically increase (around 40 percent) your risk of fatal heart attack or stroke if you take if for long periods of time. Sometimes it is even combined with opioids like codeine for pain management. Codeine itself is a phytochemical found in poppy seed. Poppy contains many alkaloids, the most important phytochemicals are morphine, noscapine, and codeine. Turmeric is even good as prebiotic. It has a positive effect on the microbiota colony in our intestines.

One more thing I want to mention is that in almost all of the cases, complete food is a better choice than extracted single phytochemical because of the phenomenon known as food synergy. Synergy means that we have two compounds they will work together much better than individual compounds combined. Two plus two equals five, if you like that analogy. This is also the reason why many of the pigments like beta carotene and lycopene in the extracted form are useless. Carrots lower the risk from cancer but beta carotene in a pill actually increases the risk. Tomatoes lower the risk of prostate cancer dramatically but lycopene increases the risk. This is very important because some supplements are more than just a waste of money and can do us harm. People might get an idea that if they don't eat enough vegetables they can get antioxidants from a pill after a nice meal of barbequed bacon. And this is not a case in all situations. There are some that can be taken as a supplement but not all of them. Curcumin from turmeric is excellent even as a supplement but for example, beta carotene and lycopene are not. If they are not packed as a whole food with thousands of other phytochemicals that work synergistically to neutralize some of the other bad effects, some of these extracted phytochemicals can do us a lot of damage. That is a reason why we always need to choose healthy food in a whole food package instead of the pills until there is extensive research done on specific phytochemicals in real clinical double-blind studies. Curcumin is well studied now and so is lycopene and so are many other phytochemicals and today we have a basic scientific knowledge of many of them. Food companies actually petitioned the FDA back in 2004 to allow them to print labels on ketchup bottles regarding lycopene and cancer risk reduction. They were denied. In that time there were a lot of mix results for tomato consumption and cancer risk because there were no real double-blind studies and people that consumed most lycopene usually got it from a pizza.

There was one man who read a bunch of unproven "quackery" about vegan diet and nutrition on the internet because he got untreatable prostate cancer. This was back in 1999. The prostate cancer metastases were spread through his body and treatment was stopped and he was sent to die. He started to eat a tablespoon of tomato paste every day because he found that in experimental research lycopene killed prostate cancer cells. At that time there were no real studies done like we have today. His PSA was 365 with metastases all over the body. He started his spoon of tomato paste in march and in may his PSA was down to 8.1 and stayed between 3 and 8 for the next 18 months. His metastases disappeared and at his last follow-up, he was completely asymptomatic and cleared from cancer (Response of hormone refractory prostate cancer to lycopene. J Urol. 2001 Aug;166(2):613). That is one of those "quackery" cases that the medical industry doesn't like that is almost too weird to be the truth. All of the billions of dollars "invested" in War on Cancer and some dude heals himself from terminal metastatic cancer with one tablespoon of tomato paste a day. He lived happily ever after. This case was well documented and could not be suppressed or ignored so in later years there were some experiments that used just lycopene in extracted form for cancer treatment. And the results were disappointing and actually, the researchers were happy that lycopene didn't cause more cancer like beta carotene in extracted form did. In some studies, it did worsen cancer. Today it is accepted that vitamin E (they always use a synthetic form of vitamin E in the testing) and selenium (supplements) cause increase risk for prostate cancer (Baseline selenium status and effects of selenium and vitamin e supplementation on prostate cancer risk. doi: 10.1093/jnci/djt456). Also does the lycopene (A randomized double-blind placebo controlled phase I-II study on clinical and molecular effects of dietary supplements in men with precancerous prostatic lesions. Chemoprevention or "chemopromotion"? doi: 10.1002/pros.22999). Why this is a case, again I can only speculate and some studies prove my point. If an antioxidant is able to turn himself into pro-oxidant and if we take them in large quantities that we were not been exposed to in our evolution, if we supplement or overdose, these antioxidants will overrun our natural detoxification mechanisms. This would not be a problem if antioxidant just give an extra electron and did nothing else but usually what they do is they want that electron back and become pro-oxidants again. And this is exactly what research shows. In low dietary doses that we would be able to get from food, the lycopene and beta carotene showed protective against cellular damage. But in higher supplemental dosage they actually caused more damage (Lycopene and beta-carotene protect against oxidative damage in HT29 cells at low concentrations but rapidly lose this capacity at higher doses. Free Radic Res. 1999 Feb;30(2):141-51).

If you want to supplement with antioxidants you would need an antioxidant that does not have the capacity to turn himself into pro-oxidant after giving its electron or if it does our body needs to have a strong detoxifying mechanism to rapidly remove it before it does damage. For example, already mentioned vitamin C becomes free radical but our kidneys just urinate it out with no need for enzymatic detoxification. In the whole food manner eating too many antioxidants could never pose any risk. Why there is such a push for extraction of these chemicals is because they can be used in medicine and charged and because the food industry will like to use them as a food additive so that they can claim health-promoting properties to unhealthy food items. We would probably have phytochemically fortified meat and bacon and ice-creams in the future. They already tried to do this with meat but they failed because again these phytochemicals are just pigments so when they try to use some of them it always stains the meat and other products giving them unnatural color or a nasty taste. This is a problem that the food industry is trying to solve. And if they solve it, and we get health-promoting bacon still there is one thing that cannot be replicated and that is food synergy. In this study, they researched exactly that, combined synergy of carotenoids (The anti-cancer effects of carotenoids and other phytonutrients resides in their combined activity. doi: 10.1016/j.abb.2015.02.018).

"Epidemiological studies have consistently shown that regular consumption of fruits and vegetables is strongly associated with reduced risk of developing chronic diseases, such as cancer. It is now accepted that the actions of any specific phytonutrient alone do not explain the observed health benefits of diets rich in fruits and vegetables as nutrients that were taken alone in clinical trials did not show consistent preventive effects. Indeed, synergistic inhibition of prostate and mammary cancer cell growth was evident when using combinations of low concentrations of various carotenoids or carotenoids with retinoic acid and the active metabolite of vitamin-D. We found that combinations of several carotenoids (e.g., lycopene, phytoene and phytofluene), or carotenoids and polyphenols (e.g., carnosic acid and curcumin) and/or other compounds (e.g., vitamin E) synergistically inhibit the androgen receptor activity and activate the EpRE/ARE system. The activation of EpRE/ARE was up to four-fold higher than the sum of the activities of the single ingredients, a robust hallmark of synergy."

It is only when they combined low doses of lycopene, phytoene, and phytofluene three phytochemicals that were found in tomatoes that they get a measurable result. Both three were tested in the low non-effective dose and as expected they did not show any clinical effect on their own. But when combined they did show measurable effect although the same low non-effective doses were used. Then when they combined curcumin with tomato extract and with vitamin E the result was suppressed tumor growth by 70 percent. That is significant suppression. Individually it was around 5 percent each, with vitamin E showing no result at all. The result of studies like this is crucial for nutrition. What studies like this show is that we need to eat health-promoting antioxidant-rich whole food and not just that. We need to have a variety of foods on our plates. Also, it has been shown that different phytochemicals bind to different receptors and different proteins in our body (Target molecules of food phytochemicals: food science bound for the next dimension doi: 10.1039/c2fo10274a). Every single phytochemical has a different receptor. There are a number of these receptors identified. EGCg, for example, is a main phytochemical in green tea and it has its own receptor. There are different binding proteins for phytochemicals in onions, grapes, broccoli, apples, oranges and as time goes science will identify more and more receptors for thousands of different phytochemicals. An antioxidant is antioxidant in a molecular sense but in our bodies, they will exert a different mode of action by binding to different receptors. We need to have a variety of foods on our plates. If we eat just meat, eggs, dairy, and refined sugar and fat in 100 different varieties our health will deteriorate. There are no phytochemical requirements for labeling in the food items. There is no phytochemical RDA. Phytochemicals are not vitamins. If we look at Fanta and orange juice the orange juice will be even worse in the amount of sugar that is in it. But because there is no labeling the whole list of phytochemicals is missing. So far the medical industry has done little to educate people in the importance of phytochemicals and research like this was only meant for a small group of scientist that are trying to develop different drugs based on them. Then that phytochemicals will be prescribed as a medicine. Medical doctors like to talk a lot about prevention but that all comes down to weight management and maybe some exercise and maybe some refined food avoidance. The real education is hard to find and even MD's themselves are deprived of nutritional education in college. What science is saying is basically what most of the people know already instinctively or by folk traditions.

Plants are good for health and we should eat our fruits and veggies and avoid greasy sausages. The problem is that we don't want to do it. We want greasy sausage with a beer. And even if we do eat vegetables, not all vegetables are made equal. If we have to compare kale with cucumbers, the kale is a clear win. Some plants have more phytochemicals and are much more nutritious than the others. The problem is that usually even when people chose fruits and vegetables, they chose the ones that are less nutritious. Potatoes, cucumbers, green lettuce, bananas instead of kale, spinach, berries, and spices. When we look at the antioxidant potential of different pigments the question arises, what is the most powerful and most health-promoting off them all? We know that food synergy plays a role and that we should eat them all but also, we know that some plants are much better than others and that some pigments are much more potent than the others. So, from yellow to orange to red, what is the strongest of them all? What is the healthiest plant?

The answer is red pigment astaxanthin in a special type of microscopic algae that we would never be able to consume in higher amounts in our normal diet. These types of algae have developed a defensive mechanism to combat UV radiation because they were exposed to sunlight during the entire day in areas where there is heavy UV radiation. The richest commercial source for natural astaxanthin is freshwater microscopic algae Haematococcus pluvialis. These microscopic algae Haematococcus pluvialis, when exposed to strong light or when any other environmental stressor is present like for example increase in salinity, will start to accumulate a bright red carotenoid pigment that is known as astaxanthin. It is a very well-researched molecule. So far there are more than 3000 studies done on it both in vitro and in vivo. It is a carotenoid same as lycopene or beta carotene. The big difference is that it is the most powerful pigment known in science. It is much more potent than curcumin for example. It is 6000 times more potent than vitamin C and 550 times more potent than vitamin E, 5000 times more powerful than green tea, 800 times that of coenzyme Q10, 200 times that of polyphenols, 150 times that of anthocyanins (water-soluble blue pigments in berries), and 75 times that of α-Lipoic acid (Quenching activities of common hydrophilic and lipophilic antioxidants against singlet oxygen using chemiluminescence detection system. Carotenoid Science. 2007;11(6):16–20). Like other carotenoids, it is oil-soluble so that means it will accumulate in tissues. In nature it will accumulate in a food chain starting with animals that consume these types of algae. Red trout, salmon, red sea bream, flamingos, shrimps, krill, crab, lobsters all are born white. Flamingos will become red from the effects of astaxanthin accumulation in their tissues. When shrimps and other crustaceans eat this type of algae, they will accumulate this pigment and their shells will become red. As the biomagnification process happens in the food chain, the level of astaxanthin and color becomes more concentrated as it moves up creating the beautiful reds and pinks we see in fish such as salmon and in marine birds like flamingos. That nice red meat of salmon is nothing more than astaxanthin accumulation. In wild salmon, the amount of accumulated astaxanthin is in the range from 20 to 40 mg/kg of body weight. Another unique characteristic is that it is able to pass the blood-brain barrier and also retina and will accumulate in the brain and in the eyes. When examined the xanthophylls (yellow pigments, one of two major divisions of the carotenoid group which includes astaxanthin, lutein, and others) accounted for 66-77% of total carotenoids in all brain regions examined (Carotenoid, tocopherol, and retinol concentrations in elderly human brain. J Nutr Health Aging. 2004;8(3):156-62).

What this also means is that once assimilated it will remain in the cells offering long-lasting protection. Water-soluble antioxidants could not do that because they do not have the means to remain in the body. The problem is that our body is not just water or fat. It is both so to provide overall protection we need both of them. Ideally, we would consume water-soluble antioxidants in every meal during our evolution from whole plant foods so that was not an issue in the past. Today we eat animal products, oil, and refined sugar. What we need today is an oil-soluble antioxidant that can accumulate in the cells but will also provide protection in other parts of our cells that are not made out of fat. And that is exactly what this pigment can do. It is unique in that matter that is both oil and water-soluble. This is not 100 percent correct but it is sort of truth. It is an oil-soluble antioxidant but it is a very long molecule that when integrated into a cell membrane the end of that molecule will stick out of the cell membrane into the watery parts of the cells. So, although it is oil soluble the shape of the molecule will allow for it to provide protection in both parts of the cells in fats and in the water. And will go through the entire body including the brain. The molecular structure also enables it to quench free radicals at the polar end groups, while the double bonds of its middle segment remove high-energy electrons. These unique chemical properties explain some of its features, particularly a higher antioxidant activity than other carotenoids (Astaxanthin: a review of its chemistry and applications. Crit Rev Food Sci Nutr. 2006;46(2):185-96). In addition, astaxanthin protects the redox state and functional integrity of mitochondria. It is extremely strong, it is a universal antioxidant (both oil and water-soluble), it passes through the blood brain barrier and one more thing the most important of them all. It can never turn itself into pro-oxidant. After it gives all of its electrons it does no damage to DNA. Astaxanthin cannot become pro-oxidant, it just gives electrons and leaves so there is no danger in taking it. It is a molecule that is almost perfect in its design. It offers complete and lasting protection against oxidation and toxins. Everything that other pigments do like curcumin, astaxanthin will do as well except it can accumulate and is much stronger.

Besides this, there is one more benefit. There are three main enzymes that our body produces to fight free radicals. These are superoxide dismutase, catalase, and glutathione peroxidase. In studies, both three were significantly upregulated in irradiated cells in the presence of astaxanthin (Astaxanthin attenuates total body irradiation-induced hematopoietic system injury in mice via inhibition of oxidative stress and apoptosis. doi: 10.1186/s13287-016-0464-3). Therefore, it exerts significant antioxidant activities not only via direct radical scavenging but also by upregulating our own body defenses. It activates the cellular antioxidant defense system through modulation of the Nrf2 pathway. Nrf2 is a protein that regulates the expression of antioxidant proteins that is triggered by injury and inflammation. Several synthetic drugs that stimulate the Nrf2 pathway are currently being tested for the treatment of diseases that are caused by oxidative stress. Astaxanthin does this much more than any other antioxidant tested so far. Curcumin has the potential to stimulate only catalase. Astaxanthin is even more potent in this regard than curcumin. Also, so far there are no negative side effects associated with it that were ever reported. The only one I can think of would be its potential to neutralize the enzyme 5-alpha-reductase (5αR) in the body to some extent. That is the enzyme that turns testosterone into DHT (dihydrotestosterone). It can possibly lower the androgenicity in a human body by lowering DHT levels and increasing testosterone levels meaning it can protect the prostate and slow down the balding in men. Boosting testosterone levels can help with muscle mass preservation in elderly people. This also helps in cases of prostate enlargement and prostate cancer. It is also a good supplement for bodybuilding as well. There was a study that investigated the testosterone boosting supplement that contained astaxanthin and saw palmetto berry extract. A study examined the effect of astaxanthin on levels of dihydrotestosterone (DHT), testosterone, and estradiol (An open label, dose response study to determine the effect of a dietary supplement on dihydrotestosterone, testosterone and estradiol levels in healthy males. doi: 10.1186/1550-2783-5-12). These three hormones can have a role in the development of an enlarged prostate and prostate cancer as well as andropause (male menopause). Investigators gave a supplement that contained both astaxanthin and saw palmetto berry extract for 14 days. The analysis showed a significant increase in testosterone and a significant decrease in DHT and also a significant decline in estradiol as well. Because testosterone is a base hormone that enzymes in the body convert to DHT and estrogen usually if you block conversion to DHT you can expect a rise of estradiol. Because of xenoestrogens and high dairy consumption levels of estrogen are elevated in most of the population. Astaxanthin lowers DHT and lowers estrogen and boosts testosterone. All of the improvements in hormone levels seen in this study bode well for men and prostate health and also male pattern baldness and exercise and bodybuilding and even other androgenic problems like acne vulgaris. But it can also potentially lower the libido. There are no reports found on this so this is just anecdotal right now. If you already taking some of the enzyme 5-alpha-reductase blockers like finasteride for hair loss or dutasteride for prostate enlargement you can still add astaxanthin to your list of supplements but keep taking your medication as well. So far there are no real clinical studies for hair loss prevention using this pigment so I don't know how potent it is regarding this issue.

It all started when some researches got the idea that they can use astaxanthin in a sunscreen lotion as a topical product. The reasoning was if it is strong pigment and if it absorbs UV radiation and protects algae from the Sun then it will do the same thing for our skin if applied topically. They got much more then they hoped for. This pigment offered the photoprotective, antioxidant, and anti-inflammatory effects providing it to be much more beneficial. Free radical damage is what in reality destroys our skin and leads to skin aging. The mechanisms of both internal or external (photo-) aging include the generation of reactive oxygen species via oxidative metabolism and exposure to Sun ultraviolet light. The process of skin aging in a first step involves damage to DNA caused by free radicals, then comes the inflammatory response and the generation of matrix metalloproteinases that degrade collagen and elastin in the dermal skin layer (Oxidation events and skin aging. doi: 10.1016/j.arr.2015.01.001). It has been shown that astaxanthin in the skin will act on several different pathways of the oxidative stress cascade (Preventive effect of dietary astaxanthin on UVA-induced skin photoaging in hairless mice. doi: 10.1371/journal.pone.0171178). Besides UVA protection its protective role will slow down the DNA damage of the skin and increase the collagen production and will contribute to skin rejuvenation and appearance and in skin diseases. It was shown that it will help in a wide range of skin conditions where inflammation plays a role such as psoriasis and atopic dermatitis and will also help with excessive dryness and pruritus. Like glutathione, it will lighten the skin and the eyes and will help with hyperpigmentation suppression, melanin synthesis, and photo-aging inhibition. It will increase the rate of healing of injuries, skin irritation, and tumor incidence (Effective inhibition of skin cancer, tyrosinase, and antioxidative properties by astaxanthin and astaxanthin esters from the green alga Haematococcus pluvialis. doi: 10.1021/jf304609j). And for cosmetic purposes besides already mentioned effects, it was shown that it will reduce wrinkle formation almost at the level of retinol creams (Cosmetic benefits of astaxanthin on humans subjects. Acta Biochim Pol. 2012;59(1):43-7). In this study they gave 6mg of astaxanthin as an oral supplementation plus a topical cream and at the 8 weeks mark the subjects showed significant improvements in skin condition in all layers, corneocyte layer, epidermis, basal layer, and dermis. "Astaxanthin derived from the microalgae, Haematococcus Pluvialis showed improvements in skin wrinkle (crow's feet at week-8), age spot size (cheek at week-8), elasticity (crow's feet at week-8), skin texture (cheek at week-4), moisture content of corneocyte layer (cheek in 10 dry skin subjects at week-8) and corneocyte condition (cheek at week-8)." This is a clinical trial, not just some "alternative medicine". For skin so far this is maybe the best thing that nature has to offer. It lightens the skin and removes hyperpigmentation, it will protect the skin from UV radiation and free radical damage, it will reduce the wrinkles and increase elasticity and it will give you a "golden glow" like beta carotene. It is not just astaxanthin that does this, there are many other dietary antioxidant sources including polyphenols and carotenoids but astaxanthin has some unique properties and is the strongest of them all. Comparative studies examining the photoprotective effects of carotenoids have demonstrated that astaxanthin is a superior antioxidant, having greater antioxidant capacity than canthaxanthin and β-carotene in human dermal fibroblasts. That is the reason why there is so much research into it. People especially ladies always ask me what regimen I recommend for skin rejuvenation. It starts with a healthy diet and lifestyle but on top of that astaxanthin supplementation with micro-needling and with retinol cream can improve a skin condition visibly. The skin has an unlimited amount of stem cells so you can do a micro-needling with no problems and also retinol will increase cell turnover and astaxanthin will protect the skin and will increase collagen production. The only side effect that is possible if you overdo it because it accumulates in the skin is that you might go past the "golden glow" into a carotenemia. So far there is no actual case reported of astaxanthin induced carotenemia except some anecdotal reports of skin turning pink in between the fingers and palms. You will have to take substantial amounts of this pigment to stain your skin in a more visible manner but theoretically, it is possible. It does accumulate and it does have a strong red color. This is a reason why as a sunscreen product, it failed. Not in research, it has strong ultraviolet absorbing properties but as a skin product, it failed. When applied to the skin as a cream it has a red color. Putting something that looks like ketchup on your skin is not consumer friendly. We also need to keep in mind that there is nothing unique about astaxanthin except its potency and if we want to protect our skin from solar radiation, we could also do it by consuming an adequate amounts of other antioxidants from food. For example, there was a line of studies that proved that alcohol consumption decreases the protection efficiency from antioxidants and that increases the risk from sunburn (Alcohol consumption decreases the protection efficiency of the antioxidant network and increases the risk of sunburn in human skin. doi: 10.1159/000343908). This is because alcohol is a pro-inflammatory toxin that burns up the body's antioxidant defense. "The results showed a significant decrease in the carotenoid concentration in the skin and the MED after alcohol consumption, but no significant decrease after a combined intake of alcohol and orange juice."

One other area where astaxanthin has more to offer than other antioxidants is in brain protective properties. Unlike many other antioxidants, astaxanthin crosses the blood-brain barrier and accumulates in the brain. These features have led experts to label astaxanthin a natural brain food. Astaxanthin also directly combats the oxidative impact of abnormal proteins in both Alzheimer's and Parkinson's diseases. Besides this, it is an excellent supplement to combat age related cognitive decline. The nervous system is rich in both unsaturated fats (which are prone to oxidation much more than saturated fats, regular fat you see in your abdomen) and iron (that can easily oxidize and is very reactive). These, together with the intense metabolic activity and rich blood supply with a lot of blood vessels, make tissues particularly susceptible to oxidative damage. The brain consumes 20 percent of all calories that we eat and 20 percent of oxygen as well. Keep in mind that the weight of the entire brain in humans is around three pounds. The problem with the brain is that it has to protect itself from toxins and unwanted chemicals much more than the rest of the body because neural cells are very sensitive and need to have a pristine environment to work properly hence there is a blood brain barrier that keeps a lot of bad stuff out. Only two of the 20 or so dietary carotenoids, carotenoids circulating within the blood, lutein, and zeaxanthin, are typically found in the retina. At the same time, they are found in millimolar concentrations (the highest accumulation of carotenoids in the body). The retina is part of the central nervous system. Not only are lutein and zeaxanthin in ocular tissue at high amounts, but their exclusive presence also makes it clear that they are concentrated via some active mechanism. The brain, like the retina, appears to accumulate xanthophylls not simply through passive diffusion but actively because that is the only possible way to explain high concentrations of lutein and zeaxanthin in the retina. In the rest of the brain lutein is also a dominant carotenoid. When you have a low consumption of lutein and other carotenoids it will increase the cognitive decline (Low macular pigment optical density is associated with lower cognitive performance in a large, population-based sample of older adults doi: 10.1016/j.neurobiolaging.2013.05.00) and especially if you have low lutein consumption that will increase age-related macular degeneration (The Effect of Lutein on Eye and Extra-Eye Health, doi: 10.3390/nu10091321). Pigments create the color by absorbing and reflecting the different wavelengths of visible light. Lutein has the ability to filter the blue light, thus reducing phototoxic damage to photoreceptor cells in the retina. Lutein intake varies and depends on vegetable consumption. Low habitual consumption of fruit and green leafy vegetables is one of the risk factors for increasing the rate of age-related macular degeneration. Same as lutein, astaxanthin is also found to slow down age-related macular degeneration and glaucoma. These two carotenoids are very important because these are the primary carotenoids that saturate our brain. Eating high amounts of antioxidants is beneficial but if we strictly talk about the brain and eye health, these two are the main ones. In addition to protection, the xanthophylls may serve other functions in brain tissue that range from epigenetic regulation to cellular communication. Both astaxanthin, lutein and zeaxanthin are xanthophylls. But be careful, there was one reported case of a woman that had developed crystals in the retina after excessive lutein supplementation. Lutein as a supplement also has shown an increase in lung cancer risk (Long-term use of beta-carotene, retinol, lycopene, and lutein supplements and lung cancer risk: results from the VITamins And Lifestyle (VITAL) study. doi: 10.1093/aje/kwn409). In the study use of supplemental beta-carotene, retinol, and lutein supplements were associated with a significantly elevated risk of total lung cancer. This is so far just association but until more research is done, I will suggest whole food sources. In foods, lutein is found in green leafy vegetables. Kale and spinach have the highest amount. There is no lutein in animal products. There are carotenoids in egg yolk but the amount of lutein in kale, for example is 39,550 micrograms per 100 grams and in whole egg 353 micrograms per 100 grams. It is much better to get it from a whole food source but if you want to supplement you should be careful of crystal formations in the eyes and increase in cancer risk. Also, supplemental lutein has proven to be less effective than the whole food source because in a whole food source there are thousands of different phytochemicals that work in synergy. In this study (Bioavailability of natural carotenoids in human skin compared to blood. doi: 10.1016/j.ejpb.2010.06.004) researchers looked at how effective is a kale extract at increasing carotenoid concentration in the skin and there was a significant increase after kale supplementation. Then they compared the skin concentration with supplemental lycopene and lutein and a mix of carotenoids in a pill form. None of them worked. Only whole food extracts worked. They concluded that: "The higher increase in the skin may possibly be caused by the fact that the antioxidant substances in a skin act as a network, protecting each other against degradation, caused by free radicals.... vegetables, fruit, and natural extracts, which contain a cocktail of different carotenoids, or in general antioxidants protect tissues such as the skin more efficiently than high doses of single synthetic carotenoids. This indicates that antioxidants in skin protect each other in an antioxidative network."

Astaxanthin however, does not suffer from this effect probably because of its potency. It is a single phytochemical that microalgae use, or the primal phytochemical that microalgae use with the potent effects just on its own. So far it is shown to be effective and a safe product. In research in vivo in mice and in clinical trials in humans beside anti-apoptotic, anti-inflammatory and antioxidant effects, it showed potential to promote or maintain neural plasticity and to increase the rate of neurogenesis, the rate of creation of new neurons from stem cells in the hippocampus (Neuroprotective mechanisms of astaxanthin: a potential therapeutic role in preserving cognitive function in age and neurodegeneration, doi: 10.1007/s11357-017-9958-x). Besides protecting the brain, skin, and eyes astaxanthin does everything that other antioxidants do as well, but these are more unique characteristics of this pigment. Besides this, it does all the same things as curcumin even at a higher rate because it is more potent and it accumulates in the cells. It also has cancer fighting effects, protects the cholesterol from oxidizing and improves its profile and protects cardiovascular health and this include stroke prevention as well, boosts immune system, helps with infertility, helps with diabetes, helps with wounds, burns, ulcers, and sores, protects against influenza and bacterial inflammation, helps with autoimmune diseases and other inflammatory diseases, helps with inflammation in the liver, overall liver functioning, and non-alcoholic fatty liver disease, helps alleviate menopausal symptoms, can help reduce pain symptoms and inflammation related to rheumatoid arthritis and carpal tunnel syndrome. I won't analyze all of the studies, there are more than 3000 of them so far but I will say that the benefit it provides with no real side-effects makes this one of the most health-promoting molecules science has ever found. It is the strongest universal antioxidant that nature has to offer. If you don't have any disease it is still a beneficial supplement for life extension.

It prolongs longevity by protecting DNA from damage and by increasing and regulating autophagy, a self-eating mechanism of damaged cells and cellular repair that our body does when we go into fasting mode (Astaxanthin Modulation of Signaling Pathways That Regulate Autophagy. doi: 10.3390/md17100546). When we lower the rate of oxidation in the body we live longer because there is no need for DNA repair. Every time DNA splits it halves telomers in half and when there are no telomeres there is no splitting only death. By protecting DNA, we prolong life. If there is an unlimited amount of stem cells that our body can produce, we will never die. Because there isn't, the only thing we can do is to slow down the oxidation. It is even a good supplement for bodybuilding and athletes in general. And it is not on a doping substance ban list. It increases physical strength and endurance and minimizes muscle recovery time following exertion (Astaxanthin in Exercise Metabolism, Performance and Recovery: A Review, doi: 10.3389/fnut.2017.00076). When we exercise there is inflammation in the muscles due to the overproduction of the free radicals due to the high rate of oxygen consumption. Heavy breathing exists due to the increase in demand for energy. Because of this, protein, lipid, and nucleic molecules can become damaged due to an overproduction of reactive oxygen and nitrogen species. To prevent this a supplementing with strong antioxidants like astaxanthin has become a strategy for many professional athletes and active health-conscious individuals. It was a big debate until studies have been done on an issue does the prevention and lowering of this type of damage actually negate all benefits from exercise. It was believed that this damage to the muscles is actually what triggers adaptations and muscle growth and all other benefits that we have from exercise. So, it is not exercising that is healthy, it is recovery. It is a concept known as hormesis, where low exposure to the damaging agent in the first phase has a favorable biological response do to the rump up organism immune system following by higher dose inhibition. Plants that are sprayed with low doses of herbicides that are not enough to kill them have much more phytochemicals in them as a defensive response to the toxin. Or if we consume a high amount of antioxidants before exercise, will we prevent an adaptation response? The theory proposed back in 1999 was that taking excessive amounts of antioxidant rich foods and antioxidants in the extracted form will interrupt and undermine this adaptation by preventing oxidative damage in the first place. In professional sport, they feared that eating antioxidant rich food may increase recovery but prevent adaptation and by that prevent the increase in endurance and strength. In the bodybuilding world, they theorized that people who want to build muscle need to avoid any antioxidant rich food in excessive amounts or supplements especially before training in the gym.

Vitamin C has been found to do this in high doses above 1 gram (Effect of vitamin C supplements on physical performance. doi: 10.1249/JSR.0b013e31825e19cd). It reduced the negative effects of exercise-induced oxidation, including muscle damage, immune dysfunction, and fatigue. But at the same time mediated beneficial training adaptations and impaired sports performance substantially possibly by reducing mitochondrial biogenesis. In some other studies it didn't show a negative effect but this just shows how much individual this result is. If you already have high antioxidant consumption adding vitamin C will be excessive but if you are a smoker it might not be. There is no clear answer here. Doses of 200 to 400mg of vitamin C consumed through five or more servings of fruit and vegetables may be sufficient to reduce oxidative stress and provide other health benefits without impairing training adaptations. One beneficial aspect of exercise is an increase in insulin sensitivity and ameliorating type 2 diabetes. In this study researchers tested does a high rate of supplemental antioxidants have an effect on exercise induced increase in insulin sensitivity (Antioxidants prevent health-promoting effects of physical exercise in humans. doi: 10.1073/pnas.0903485106). Subjects were on a 4-week exercise regimen and 1 gram of vitamin C and 400 IU of vitamin E daily and then the insulin sensitivity was measured. Also, muscle biopsies were done for gene expression analyses as well as plasma samples. The goal was to compare changes and potential influence of antioxidant vitamins (vitamin C and E) on exercise effects.

"Exercise increased parameters of insulin sensitivity only in the absence of antioxidants in both previously untrained and pretrained individuals. Molecular mediators of endogenous ROS defense (superoxide dismutases 1 and 2; glutathione peroxidase) were also induced by exercise, and this effect too was blocked by antioxidant supplementation. Consistent with the concept of mitohormesis, exercise-induced oxidative stress ameliorates insulin resistance and causes an adaptive response promoting endogenous antioxidant defense capacity. Supplementation with antioxidants may preclude these health-promoting effects of exercise in humans."

"Physical exercise exerts numerous favorable effects on general health and specifically has been shown to improve glucose metabolism in the insulin-resistant state. This effect may be independent of exercise-related changes in body mass. Moreover, physical exercise has been shown to be effective in preventing type 2 diabetes in high-risk individuals and may be even more effective than the most widely used anti-diabetic drug, metformin. These results indicate that antioxidants severely impair the insulin-sensitizing effects of physical exercise as quantified by several measures and that this effect occurs irrespective of previous training status. In the present study, physical exercise resulted in a strongly increased expression of superoxide dismutase 1 and 2 and glutathione peroxidase in previously untrained and previously trained, antioxidant naïve individuals, whereas pretreatment with antioxidants prevented this induction. Similar while less pronounced effects were observed for catalase."

"Taken together, we find that antioxidant supplements prevent the induction of molecular regulators of insulin sensitivity and endogenous antioxidant defense by physical exercise. Consistent with the concept of mitohormesis, we propose that transiently increased levels of oxidative stress reflect a potentially health-promoting process at least in regards to prevention of insulin resistance and type 2 diabetes mellitus."

Today this theory is partially accepted. Preventing oxidative damage in the muscle does not affect any positive adaptation we have from exercising if we have a normal intake of antioxidants that are in line with what we have been eating during our evolution. It is exactly the opposite. It speeds up the recovery and increases protein synthesis and increases endurance. If we talk about antioxidants that we get from a whole good source. But what happens when we take unnatural supraphysiological doses of extracted antioxidants or antioxidant supplements? When we exercise free radicals are formed and our body increases our own antioxidants or in other words, it increases already mention antioxidant enzymes (i.e., superoxide dismutase, catalase, and glutathione peroxidase). In a situation where exercise is too vigorous, however, excessive production of free radicals can overwhelm the endogenous antioxidant defense system, causing a state of oxidative stress. If our own body defense is overrun it will have potentially detrimental impacts on normal physiological function. Dietary antioxidants have the potential to supplement our own internal defense mechanisms and prevent damage and increase performance and recovery as a result. Exercise has shown to be protective because it will actually increase the production of these three enzymes in the long run as an adaptive mechanism. The main benefit of all that running on a treadmill is just antioxidant protection. So, if antioxidants can block the main benefit from exercise and that is increasing in our own antioxidant production then consuming some high antioxidant rich food can have the same beneficial cardiovascular effects as doing the cardio itself.

In one study from Japan (Curcumin ingestion and exercise training improve vascular endothelial function in postmenopausal women. doi: 10.1016/j.nutres.2012.09.002), researchers compared rigorous physical exercise with a tablespoon of turmeric effects on endothelial function. Endothelial cells are cells that form a line in the interior surface of blood vessels. Impaired endothelial function is a first sign in the development of cardiovascular diseases and the development of atherosclerosis. It is found in people who smoke or have high blood pressure, diabetes, thrombosis, coronary artery disease, hypercholesterolemia. In the study, subjects had to do aerobic exercise training for 8 weeks in the duration of 60 minutes every day or take a teaspoon of turmeric. Both groups improved their endothelial function significantly. Turmeric group showed the level of improvement even slightly better than the exercise group. So, 60 minutes of exercise is the same as one small tablespoon of turmeric. This, however, doesn't mean you should stop exercising. There is a wide range of benefits from exercise besides an increase in antioxidant protection that I already wrote about in the first book of the series. Ideally, we should do both. It is the stress that triggers our body to adapt by increasing the production of superoxide dismutase, catalase, and glutathione peroxidase. For example, marathon runners will have increase in DNA damage during the race but six days later they will actually have much less DNA damage then if they didn't run at all thanks to the increase in our own body internal antioxidant defenses (Endurance exercise results in DNA damage as detected by the comet assay. Free Radic Biol Med. 2004 Apr 15;36(8):966-75). By stressing the body, we reap benefits in the long run.

Taking antioxidant supplements have the potential to negate this effect. But what about the whole food source of antioxidants? There was a line of studies that looked into the effects of consumption of high antioxidant food sources on athletic performance. Anthocyanin flavonoid-rich blueberries, for example, were found to decrease inflammatory muscle damage and sourness, cherries were found to speed up recovery, same with dark chocolate, tomato juice was found to improve performance level. Antioxidants in fruit, vegetables, and even beans were found to be potent inhibitors of xanthine oxidase activity (Inhibition of xanthine oxidase by flavonoids. Biosci Biotechnol Biochem. 1999 Oct;63(10):1787-90). Xanthine oxidase is the main free radical that is formed during exercise but it is also involved in the pathogenesis of several diseases such as vascular disorders, cancer, and gout. For example, a single serving of watercress for two months entirely prevents exercise-induced DNA damage (Acute and chronic watercress supplementation attenuates exercise-induced peripheral mononuclear cell DNA damage and lipid peroxidation. doi: 10.1017/S0007114512000992). This is well known in professional sport. High-level athletes have their diets optimized by nutritional experts in order to increase their performance. Food that increases endurance and strength and decreases recovery time is in a sense a "holy grail" of sports nutrition. But the question still remains, if vitamin C and E in supplemental form block adaptation will the antioxidant rich food do the same? There was a line of studies that looked into this question as well. In this study from 2008, the effects of black currant extract consumption on counteracting the positive effects of the exercise was examined (Short-term blackcurrant extract consumption modulates exercise-induced oxidative stress and lipopolysaccharide-stimulated inflammatory responses. doi: 10.1152/ajpregu.90740.2008). The result was as expected. The high antioxidant potency of the anthocyanins rich blackcurrant extract suppressed exercise-induced oxidative stress. At the same time, it boosted the positive effects of exercise as well. A similar result was obtained in other similar studies. The purpose of this study (Effect of lemon verbena supplementation on muscular damage markers, proinflammatory cytokines release and neutrophils' oxidative stress in chronic exercise. doi: 10.1007/s00421-010-1684-3) was to determine the effect of moderate antioxidant supplementation (lemon verbena extract) in healthy male volunteers that followed a 90 minutes running eccentric exercise protocol for 21 days. They wanted to see does exercise induced adaptation depends on antioxidant rich food sources, in this case, lemon verbena extract. The conclusion was: "Intense running exercise for 21 days induced an antioxidant response in neutrophils of the trained male through the increase of the antioxidant enzymes catalase, glutathione peroxidase, and glutathione reductase. Supplementation with moderate levels of an antioxidant lemon verbena extract did not block this cellular adaptive response and also reduced exercise-induced oxidative damage of proteins and lipids in neutrophils and decreased myeloperoxidase activity. Moreover, lemon verbena supplementation maintained or decreased the level of serum transaminases activity indicating the protection of muscular tissue. Exercise induced a decrease of interleukin-6 and interleukin-1β levels after 21 days measured in basal conditions, which was not inhibited by antioxidant supplementation. Therefore, moderate antioxidant supplementation with lemon verbena extract protects neutrophils against oxidative damage, decreases the signs of muscular damage in chronic running exercise without blocking the cellular adaptation to exercise." It protected the muscle, boost the performance and recovery and at the same time did not affect positive adaptation to exercise. Best of both worlds. This is a moderately powerful antioxidant that might not be strong enough to suppress adaptation, but what about something stronger. What about curcumin for example? We already know that one teaspoon of it has the same positive effect on the cardiovascular system as 60 minutes of exercise. What if you exercise and take curcumin together? Will it negate the adaptation, it is a very strong antioxidant? In this study (Effect of endurance exercise training and curcumin intake on central arterial hemodynamics in postmenopausal women: pilot study. doi: 10.1038/ajh.2012.24) they measured the effects of curcumin alone, exercise alone and curcumin plus exercise on arterial function. The positive effect was present in both groups with curcumin showing better results than exercise but when combined the positive effect was more than doubled then each group put together showing not just that there is no negative effect on exercise adaptation but that there is actually a significant synergistic effect. Curcumin didn't block the benefit of exercise but enhanced it. They concluded: "These findings suggest that regular endurance exercise combined with daily curcumin ingestion may reduce LV afterload to a greater extent than monotherapy with either intervention alone in postmenopausal women." The theory that taking an excessive amount of antioxidant rich foods and antioxidants in the extracted form will interrupt and undermine this adaptation by preventing oxidative damage is partially correct. When antioxidants are consumed in a whole food way as nature intended there is no undermining of adaptation. Only supplemental antioxidants like vitamin C and vitamin E have shown this effect. Whole food extracts didn't show this effect. They did block the oxidative damage to the muscles during exercise but did not block positive adaptation afterward. What about extracted astaxanthin in a supplemental form? What would its effects be?

Why vitamin C for example but not curcumin in a whole food way stop our body upregulation of antioxidant enzymes is a complicated science. It has to do with the activation of something called (Nrf2) erythroid 2-related factor 2 (Nrf2 mediates redox adaptations to exercise. doi: 10.1016/j.redox.2016.10.003). "Nrf2 is the master regulator of antioxidant defenses, a transcription factor that regulates expression of more than 200 genes. Increasing evidence indicates that Nrf2 signaling plays a key role in how oxidative stress mediates the beneficial effects of exercise. Episodic increases in oxidative stress induced through bouts of acute exercise stimulate Nrf2 activation and when applied repeatedly, as with regular exercise, leads to upregulation of endogenous antioxidant defenses and overall greater ability to counteract the damaging effects of oxidative stress."

Research utilizing animal models have identified a potential for astaxanthin to indirectly modulate the endogenous antioxidant defense system such as Nrf2 independently from exercise. It will independently activate our body defense mechanism with or without exercise. It is not just a strong universal antioxidant by itself but it also on top of that upregulates our own defensive mechanisms independently with or without exercise (Astaxanthin-rich extract from the green alga Haematococcus pluvialis lowers plasma lipid concentrations and enhances antioxidant defense in apolipoprotein E knockout mice doi: 10.3945/jn.111.142109).

"Once activated, the Nrf2–ARE signaling pathway initiates the transcription of several genes and enzymes capable of upregulating our own antioxidant response to an oxidative stressor, potentially implicating Nrf2 in the beneficial effects of exercise. Similarly, phytochemicals can also stimulate the activation of the Nrf2–ARE pathway, a process that may occur through the modification of different cysteine residues to those targeted through exercise, suggesting a potential synergism between exercise and phytochemicals in the upregulation of antioxidant defense. Although a specific mechanism of action has yet to be elucidated, research conducted in animal models report increases in Nrf2 expression, alongside the upregulation of endogenous antioxidant enzymes, including superoxide dismutase, catalase and glutathione peroxidase, following astaxanthin administration" (Astaxanthin in Exercise Metabolism, Performance and Recovery: A Review. doi: 10.3389/fnut.2017.00076).

Astaxanthin, curcumin, whole food, and whole-food extras do not block exercise induced adaptation but actually independently boost our own defenses through gene expression that has a different activation pathway then exercise. Only supplemental vitamin C and vitamin E block adaptation. On top of boosting our own defense and being extremely potent antioxidant just by itself, astaxanthin boosts endurance, strength, and recovery. When we start to exercise our body would start to use stored sugar (glycogen) reserves for energy. Both the liver and muscles store glycogen. If exercise is prolonged all of the glycogen stores will be utilized. If we want to increase endurance by delaying fatigue onset, we will have to find a method aimed at attenuating this depletion. When sugar is depleted our body will start to use fat as an energy source but that process is much slower than using just stored glycogen. The breakdown of fat is dependent upon the entry of long-chain fatty acids into the mitochondria to be burned as energy. This process is done by using mitochondrial CPT1 regulatory enzyme. During exercise, free radical induced oxidative damage to this enzyme can alter its function, blocking the transportation of fatty acids and consequently limiting the ability for fats to be oxidized as a viable energy source. Astaxanthin as an oil-soluble antioxidant is known to accumulate in the mitochondrial membrane and provide protection against free radical induced damage to CPT1 function (Astaxanthin improves muscle lipid metabolism in exercise via inhibitory effect of oxidative CPT I modification. Biochem Biophys Res Commun. 2008 Feb 22;366(4):892-7). It has, therefore, been hypothesized that through its function as an antioxidant, astaxanthin could protect CPT1 against oxidative damage, causing an indirect enhancement of fat metabolism in the process. In research, it was proven that astaxanthin benefits endurance through enhancing fat utilization as an energy source and consequently attenuating muscle glycogen depletion (Effects of astaxanthin supplementation on exercise-induced fatigue in mice. Biol Pharm Bull. 2006 Oct;29(10):2106-10). Besides increasing endurance in this study astaxanthin also significantly decreased fat accumulation. It is a good supplement for increasing fat utilization which means it is good for dieting and obesity and diabetes. Also, by increasing fat utilization, we will feel less hungry, have better control of our appetite, and don't have low blood sugar during dieting as well. Also, increase utilization of fat means a decrease in the utilization of muscle tissue and catabolism during dieting. Bodybuilders should love this supplement. In human trials, a similar enhancing of physical performance was reported. In amateur male cyclists, 4 weeks of astaxanthin supplementation (4 mg/day) significantly improved 20 km cycling time (Effect of astaxanthin on cycling time trial performance. doi: 10.1055/s-0031-1280779). After the exercise, there is soreness or in other words inflammation cascade. Astaxanthin is excellent for fighting inflammation. If recovery is inadequate following exercise, it may prevent recreationally active individuals and athletes from training again. Inadequate recovery may also increase risks of injury, illness and overtraining. As a result, there are different strategies that can reduce the negative effect of exercise-induced muscle damage and accelerate recovery. Astaxanthin could exert a recovery benefit through the inhibition of both pro-oxidant and pro-inflammatory intermediates. Astaxanthin supplementation (4 mg/day) was suggested to augment these reductions further, while also exerting a secondary anti-inflammatory effect through attenuating training-induced increases in serum C-reactive protein and total leukocyte and neutrophil counts (Effect of Astaxanthin Supplementation on Salivary IgA, Oxidative Stress, and Inflammation in Young Soccer Players. doi: 10.1155/2015/783761). As a sports supplement astaxanthin has more benefits. It increases endurance and strength, enhances fat utilization, supports recovery but it is also good for boosting testosterone levels as well. On top of this, it independently increases protein synthesis. In this study (Combined intake of astaxanthin, β-carotene, and resveratrol elevates protein synthesis during muscle hypertrophy in mice. doi: 10.1016/j.nut.2019.110561) the researchers wanted to measure the impact of different antioxidants on building the skeletal muscle mass and protein synthesis or in other words muscle hypertrophy. To induce atrophy in the muscle one leg of each mouse was cast for 3 weeks. After removal of the cast, the mice were fed diet for 2 weeks with supplemental β-carotene, astaxanthin, resveratrol, and all three antioxidants combined. The weight of the soleus muscle was increased in all groups to a greater extent than in the control group with the highest increase in the mixed group. The conclusion of this study is that antioxidants are a good way to go if you want to build muscle. Nonetheless, an increase in protein synthesis is far from what anabolic steroids would do so don't expect magic.

If you decide to take this supplement how much should you take? There is no clear answer. The more is usually better when we talk about antioxidant consumption from whole food sources. In supplemental form, some benefits will start as low as 4mg a day. Depending on your general quality of the diet this can be a potential starting point but the most common dose is 12mg a day. You can go safely much higher than this. If you go with higher doses not all of the astaxanthin will be utilized but it would not be excreted as well. Keep in mind that this molecule is fat-soluble and that it accumulates. The higher you go the more astaxanthin will accumulate in the tissues. Half-life is about 15 hours with a peak concentration in the blood of around 10 hours. In wild salmon, astaxanthin tissue concentration can go as high as 40mg/kg. For 80kg human that will translate into 3200mg. If you take 12mg a day that means you will go to this level of wild salmon concentration in 267 days if your body doesn't utilize any of the ingested astaxanthin and that is not the case. More realistically it would be hard to reach full body saturation with 12mg dose. It is more of the maintenance dose if you are not a smoker, and have the whole food, plant based, antioxidant rich diet. What I recommend is to start with a loading phase of 3 months of 40mg/day and then see how you feel. This would be a total of 3600mg and then you can transition to the maintenance phase. Another way is to go as long as you don't see visible signs of carotenemia before lowering the dose. This would be an individual approach that might be the most optimal one. Also, there are synthetic and natural astaxanthin. Synthetic astaxanthin is used as a food additive for farmed salmon. It is used as a tissue die to give a farmed salmon a natural looking pink color of the meat. Synthetic astaxanthin from petrochemicals and astaxanthin derived from genetically mutated phaffia yeast have never been proven beneficial and have not been proven safe for direct human consumption. One more thing to keep in mind. Because astaxanthin, beta carotene, and other carotenoids are oil-soluble the absorption is greatly increased if we consume them with food or oil (Bioavailability of astaxanthin in Haematococcus algal extract: the effects of timing of diet and smoking habits. Biosci Biotechnol Biochem. 2009 Sep;73(9):1928-32).

How strong is, for example, 12mg capsule compared to other antioxidants? Units that measure the antioxidant capacity of different substances are called ORAC. ORAC stands for Oxygen Radical Absorbance Capacity. It's a lab test developed by scientists at the National Institute of Health and Aging (NIH) that attempts to measure the total antioxidant capacity of a specific food or supplement or any substance by placing a sample in a test tube, along with certain molecules that generate free radical activity and certain other molecules that are vulnerable to oxidation. After a while, they measure how well the sample protected the vulnerable molecules from oxidation by the free radicals. The less free radical damage there is, the higher the antioxidant capacity of the test substance. With this kind of testing researchers have a way of measuring the total antioxidant capacity of different whole food items rather than the levels of specific nutrients. Because there are thousands of different phytochemicals this method of measurement detects real-life values that we will get from food with all of the synergistic effects between the various nutrients. This is also a way to measure different antioxidants in extracted form like vitamin C or vitamin E or any other unique antioxidant compounds in plants. This method of measurement is a good way of comparing the antioxidant power of different whole food items and individual substances that we can find in different supplements. One thing that we should keep in mind here is that the same food items can have different values depending on a manufacturer. If we grind, for example, cocoa bean into cocoa powder there is no protective outer layer any longer to prevent it from oxidizing. The longer it sits on an open air the more it will oxidize and the lower will the ORAC reading be. That is the reason we can see a range of different values in ORAC reading for cocoa, cinnamon or any other item that can oxidize then for example beans that can sit on a shelf for a long time without oxidizing. As soon as the item is exposed to air, oxidation starts. This is the reason why you should never consume flaxseed oil. Omega 3 oils are very prone to oxidation. If you grind flaxseeds and eat them immediately there would be a lower level of oxidation. If you like to blend something into a smoothie the level of oxidation caused by blending can destroy a large number of antioxidants in food. Vacuum blenders are a new way of blending food in order to preserve the nutrients in them. Masticating juicers that use a form of the press to extract juice will have juice with a higher antioxidant value than regular juice. That is the reason that we can see a big difference in the same food items tested because of the different methods of manufacturing. Also, some items may seem low on the ORAC scale but are actually not. For example, watermelon has relatively low value but that is because it is mostly just water. For the same reason dry fruits will have a much higher rating than the same fresh fruit because they are much more concentrated. Fresh fruit will have higher water content and therefore lower ORAC values. Spices are another example. Spices are dry and therefore will have in a gram of dry weight higher ORAC value than the same fresh herb that has higher water content. Also, we have to take into account the amounts of specific foods that we can eat. Spices are extremely potent in antioxidant capacity but we can only eat small amounts of them. One food item can be low on an ORAC scale but when we see in real life how much of that food is consumed then it might be actually a good source of antioxidants. It all depends on specific foods. We can eat a handful of walnuts with no problem but eating a handful of cloves is difficult. Per serving bases nuts have more antioxidants then cloves. But then again, nuts are full of calories. We can analyze an antioxidant per calorie consumed as well. The general rule and the main rule is that animal products including dairy, all types of meat and eggs have zero or minuscule amounts of antioxidants and are actually pro-inflammatory. Only plant foods have measurable ORAC values and not all plants are made equal.

The first database of ORAC values was released by USDA in 2007 and it covered 277 food items. Then in 2010, the research was published that took 8 years to complete and included the antioxidative value of 3149 food items (The total antioxidant content of more than 3100 foods, beverages, spices, herbs and supplements used worldwide. doi: 10.1186/1475-2891-9-3). They measured every food, every beverage, every supplement they can find. This was one of the most important studies ever done in the field of nutrition. It is important because it has real-life value for a regular person that is going to a market because it can guide regular shopping decisions we make all the time. We can search the database for every single food item but most importantly, we can get some general rules out of it. The first rule that this study found was that the average ORAC value for animal based foods is almost nothing. On average plant foods have more than 30 times more antioxidants than animal based foods. The second thing that we need to consider is that there is a wide range of values even for plant foods. It ranges from zero to 2,897,110 µmol TE/100g for the number one on the list. That is almost 3 million in value. The number one antioxidant rich food item on the planet is called Sangre de grado (Dragon's Blood). Dragon's blood is the name given to an intensely red tree sap which oozes from the Croton lechleri tree when its trunk has been cut or injured. It's native to the northwestern part of South America, primarily Columbia, Ecuador, Peru, and Bolivia. Though it is worth mentioning there is conflicting research out there as to whether or not it might have a side effect of being a mutagen. Currently, a lot more research needs to be done on its effects. In the animal kingdom, for comparison, the highest value is ox liver at 710. Actually, there is one animal kingdom food item that has much more antioxidants and that is human breast milk with a score of 2030. On average eggs are just 40, dairy 140, fish 110, meat and meat products 310 and chicken is 230. To compare let's look at the worst of the plant kingdom, cucumber raw without peel at 140, iceberg lettuce at 438 and watermelon at 142. Legumes are averaging at 480, grains at 340, vegetables 800 but then nuts and seeds have an average of 4570, berries and berry products 9860, spices and herbs 29020 and the highest category is herbal/traditional plant medicine with an average rating of 91720.

They concluded: "The results here uncover that the antioxidant content of foods varies several thousand-fold and that antioxidant rich foods originate from the plant kingdom while meat, fish and other foods from the animal kingdom are low in antioxidants. Comparing the mean value of the 'Meat and meat products' category with plant based categories, fruits, nuts, chocolate, and berries have from 5 to 33 times higher mean antioxidant content than the mean of meat products. Diets comprised mainly of animal-based foods are thus low in antioxidant content while diets based mainly on a variety of plant-based foods are antioxidant rich, due to the thousands of bioactive antioxidant phytochemicals found in plants which are conserved in many foods and beverages."

At this point in time, this line of scientific research is well established and well accepted but only in the scientific community that is doing them for the interest of the pharmaceutical industry. You will be able to find all of this on the PubMed website but outside of the narrow scientific community, nobody is talking. The regular public will hear something here and there with no real awareness. When you ask a medical establishment, they will tell a completely different story. In accepted health recommendations pushed by physicians, there is no room for antioxidants. The medical establishment doesn't want people to know this and will argue that antioxidants are of no major importance for the health and that they are not vitamins and that there is no need for RDA for antioxidant or phytochemical consumption. We don't really have public awareness of phytochemical importance and regular science will tell people everything they can just to confuse and undermine awareness. They will not talk about antioxidants, they will not enforce RDA in the food pyramid and will do anything to confuse people on purpose. They will use half-truths and actually the entire database of ORAC values had been removed from the USDA website. So how much do we need if any? The story they impose is that the body can effectively only use 3000-5000 ORAC units per day and that any more is useless. Any more than this (i.e. with mega-dosing in supplemental form or eating antioxidant rich food) seems to be of no added benefit and "excess" is most likely excreted by the kidneys. Good example of this is, for example, a statement from Dr. Ronald Prior of the US Department of Agriculture Research Service at Tufts University, Boston, Massachusetts that is quoted to have said: "A significant increase in antioxidants of 15-20% is possible by increasing consumption of fruits and vegetables, particularly those high in ORAC value. However, in order to have a significant impact on plasma and tissue antioxidant capacity one can only meaningfully increase one's daily intake by 3000-5000 ORAC units. Any greater amount is probably redundant. That is because the antioxidant capacity of the blood is tightly regulated. Thus, there is an upper limit to the benefit that can be derived from antioxidants. Taking in 25000 ORAC units at one time would be no more beneficial than taking in a fifth of that amount. The excess is simply excreted by the kidneys". They are just lying to you. There are water-soluble antioxidants that can be removed by the kidneys. The similar story is with vitamin C and that is correct. If you take too much vitamin C excess will be removed but Dr. Ronald somehow forgets about the fact that not all antioxidants are water-soluble. Oil-soluble substances cannot be removed through kidneys. Any excess of them will bioaccumulate and will offer long-lasting protection. And not just that, water-soluble antioxidants do their job of lowering inflammation and neutralizing free radicals before removal as well. I will analyze later in this chapter just how much antioxidants we really need but this recommendation by people that have Ph.D.'s and six-figure salaries are not from ignorance. They have a deliberate agenda to confuse people. They want you to give your entire income on chemotherapy and spend all of your money on drugs, therapies, animal products and other junk food. Healthy people that eat vegetables are not good customers. Because there is no "official" daily recommended intake of ORAC units, you will see various researchers suggest an optimal intake to be only 3000-5000 ORAC units per day, and many of the physicians will not recommend antioxidant rich diets at all. They will tell their patients absolutely nothing about thousands and thousands of studies done on a topic and will usually just suggest losing weight and physical exercise with a line of prescribed medicine as a standard line of treatment. And this is not by accident. Even the USDA has come up with a suggested intake of 5000 ORAC units per day. The UK FSA and the FDA recommend "5 a day" of fruit and vegetable servings, which give an approximate ORAC score of 3500. It is all just a joke and even worse, deliberate conspiracy. So, what real scientific research that is available has to say about it?

We use glucose and oxygen to create energy just for existence meaning we have a basic caloric need just for regular metabolism. Burning energy for sustenance without any other added stress or toxin creates free radicals just by itself. Oxidizing glucose to make energy is not perfect and some free radicals will form no matter what. Because of this every time we eat something during regular metabolism there will be an increase in the level of oxidation in our bloodstreams over the next few hours as our bodies metabolize the glucose for energy. This is a completely normal reaction. Not just regular metabolism but many other processes will also create a depletion of our antioxidant reserve. For example, stressful events, infections, exercise, toxins, and many other stressors. In evolutional terms, we have never eaten meat and animal products in a meaningful amount. For the last 60 million years of evolution, we have been sustaining ourselves on whole plant foods and now we have a problem. In nature sugar always comes with phytonutrients. We have evolved to expect a burst of dietary antioxidants any time we eat. But what happens when we eat refined sugar, oil and animal products? In the developed world most calories come from this type of food. Where are the expected antioxidants to prevent inflammation and DNA damage? If we don't eat phytonutrient rich plant foods with each meal, then for hours after we eat, our bodies are tipped out of balance into a pro-oxidative state, which can set us up for oxidant stress diseases and will increase a rate of DNA damage meaning we will age more rapidly. That's why we need to ideally eat antioxidant rich foods with every meal and during the entire day to sustain our antioxidant levels in the positive balance as much as we can. This is what for example British Journal of Nutrition has to say about it (Postprandial metabolic events and fruit-derived phenolics: a review of the science. doi: 10.1017/S0007114510003909). "Postprandial (fed) state is a pro-oxidant state. The postprandial period is a time of active oxidative metabolism and formation of ROS (free radicals). There is increasing evidence that the postprandial state is an important contributing factor to chronic disease. Two main questions are posed: first, what is the role of plant foods, specifically fruits rich in complex and simple phenolic compounds in postprandial metabolic management; and second, does the evidence support consuming these fruits with meals as a practical strategy to preserve health and lower risk for disease? The collected data suggest that consuming phenolic-rich fruits increases the antioxidant capacity of the blood, and when they are consumed with high fat and carbohydrate 'pro-oxidant and pro-inflammatory' meals, they may counterbalance their negative effects. Given the content and availability of fat and carbohydrate in the Western diet, regular consumption of phenolic-rich foods, particularly in conjunction with meals, appears to be a prudent strategy to maintain oxidative balance and health." To some extent, Dr. Ronald was correct. Taking in 25000 ORAC units at one time would be no more beneficial than taking in 5000 ORAC units five times a day because in seven or eight hours the excess might be excreted. We cannot just eat 10 serving of blueberries for breakfast and eat bacon rest of the day. Taking 5000 units five times a day is an optimal strategy. Or even better, taking in 25000 units five times a day. There was a line of studies done on this subject in the last 10 to 15 years. In this study (Plasma antioxidant capacity changes following a meal as a measure of the ability of a food to alter in vivo antioxidant status. J Am Coll Nutr. 2007 Apr;26(2):170-81) they looked into different studies that analyzed how much different fruit influences postprandial oxidative state. Dried plums or dried plum juice, for example, didn't alter hydrophilic (water-soluble) or lipophilic (oil soluble) antioxidant capacity which was surprising to me. Plums are one of the richest sources of antioxidants and have high ORAC value but it looks like their antioxidants in vivo might not be bioavailable. Blueberries increased both hydrophilic and lipophilic antioxidant capacity and cherries increased plasma lipophilic but not hydrophilic antioxidant capacity. The conclusion was: "We have demonstrated that consumption of certain berries and fruits such as blueberries, mixed grape, and kiwifruit, was associated with increased plasma AOC (antioxidant capacity) in the postprandial state and consumption of an energy source of macronutrients containing no antioxidants was associated with a decline in plasma AOC. Consumption of high antioxidant foods with each meal is recommended in order to prevent periods of postprandial oxidative stress." Because they believed that avoiding high fat meals is unavoidable for most of the population, meaning people will eat animal products and refined foods no matter what, the practical implication of this study in their mind was to promote consumption of fruit with high polyphenolic content with every meal or as a dessert to prevent oxidative damage correlated with postprandial oxidative state and postprandial lipemia (high levels of fat in the bloodstream). If we don't eat enough of phytonutrient rich plant foods during the day, like most of the people on the standard American diet, our bodies will be in a constant pro-oxidative state that will in a long run create many diseases. And when I say diseases, I mean real life-threatening illnesses like cancer for example. Most of the diseases of affluence are caused by a bad diet. Free radicals will oxidase fat and cholesterol in our bloodstream and that will greatly increase the risk of cardiovascular disease. Even if we don't eat an abundance of high quality phytochemical rich food, we at least should eat enough antioxidants to counteract the oxidation from the digestion of calories. To do that, researchers in the study above and in numerous other studies have calculated just how much antioxidants we need to counteract our metabolic rate.

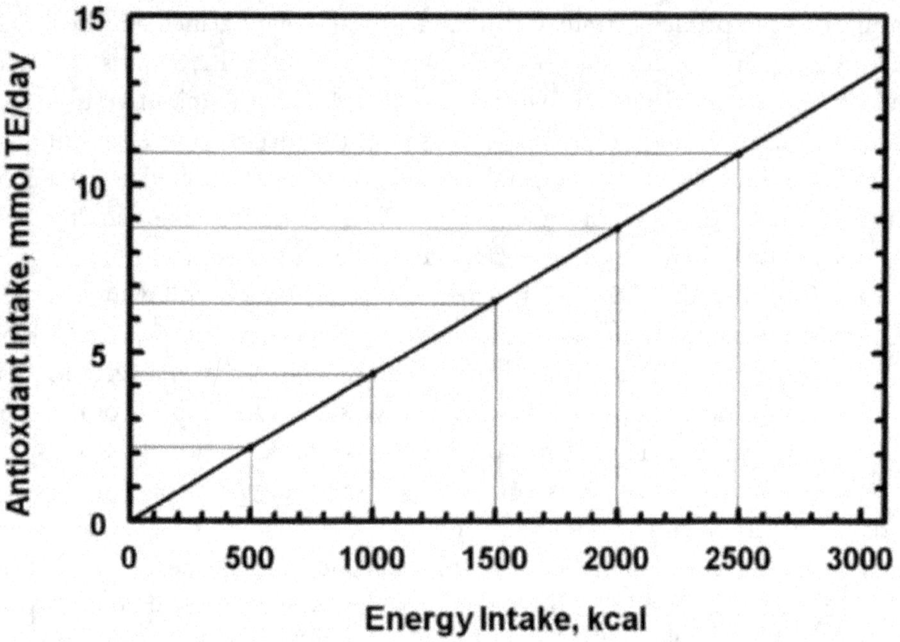

Fig. 7. Estimated antioxidant intake required (mmol/day) to prevent postprandial oxidative stress relative to energy intake (kcal).

Depending on calories we need the amount of antioxidants will vary also. For example, if you need 2500 calories for your basal metabolic rate you will need 11000 ORAC units a day. If your basal metabolism is at 1800 calories you will need 8000 ORAC units. If you burn more you will need more. This is just to counteract the metabolic oxidation. If you eat animal products, animal protein has pro-oxidative properties just by itself, you will need more. Alcohol is severely pro-inflammatory and toxic for the body. If you drink or smoke you will need more. If you have an infection or any disease you will need more. On top of that, we are all exposed to environmental toxins so depending on your individual toxic load you will need more. As you age you will need more. There is a concept known as inflame-aging. As we age, we have a decline in immune function but also immune cells of elderly people produce much more pro-inflammatory cytokines. The answer is more anti-inflammatory food sources in our diet. Ideally, we should consume all our ORAC units from whole plant-based foods during the entire day. Our daily maximum is not 3000 units or 5000 units. Our daily minimum is 8000 to 10000 just to counteract metabolism. On top of that, we should add 5000 to 10000 units more because of the toxic overload and if you are a smoker or drink alcohol or have other bad habits you should add at least 5000 to 10000 more. If you have influenza or infection or any other disease you should add much more and if you are stressed or sleep deprived you should add more also. If you want to fight against DNA damage for longevity purposes and DNA protection again you should add 5000 to 10000 more. My recommendation for optimal antioxidant RDA is between 30000 to 40000 ORAC units depending on individual lifestyle. Not 3000 to 5000 currently accepted value of recommendation by the FDA. In reality, even 3000 units is a number that most people on a standard American diet will have a hard time reaching and that is not enough, not even close. The reason the government recommends 3000 units is because in their research that will be the number that most of the people will accept because people can reach that with a couple of servings of fruits and vegetables and we don't want people to change their real dietary habits. That is not good for the business. The government slogan of "5 a Day" is for the consistent consumption of five fruits and vegetables a day supplying an average ORAC value of 2500 ORAC units. This is just a manipulation of medical science for the maintenance of the status quo. If the FDA recommended real values it would completely destroy the current food pyramid and everything the government is preaching for the last century.

But even this minuscule value that you can reach with a pinch of cinnamon is, in reality, a number that most of the people won't even reach. The sad reality is that only 5% of the U.S. population consumes 5 fruits and vegetables a day. The National Cancer Institute found that 42% of the population eats less than 2 servings a day. The average American will eat as low as 300 ORAC units in a day. Also, when you eat fruits, you need to remember that some of the phytochemicals are not resistant to heat and that in time their antioxidant value is decreasing because of the exposure to the air. For example, it is much better to buy whole flaxseeds and then grind them yourself and eat them immediately then to purchase ground flaxseeds in a store. Any antioxidant nutrients that make it through harvesting then become diminished to some extent due to the cooking, processing, preserving, packaging or just exposure to the air.

When we have a diet that is so deprived of phytochemicals and a government that wants to keep this knowledge from the general public, we have a situation where coffee had become the number one source of antioxidants. I don't want to undermine the benefits of coffee but it is not the reason that most people are drinking it. They just want caffeine high. Some of the most antioxidant-rich beverages actually are the ones that people consume regularly like coffee, tea, and red wine. The problem is that the intake of these drinks makes a significant contribution to the total amount of antioxidants consumed because the number of antioxidants consumed is minuscule. These drinks are far from potent sources of antioxidants. If you want a drink then cocoa will be a better choice. Cocoa is the most balanced product in terms of antioxidants since it contains both water-soluble and lipid-soluble antioxidants and it is very potent. How much is in coffee? The antioxidant value of brewed Arabica coffee, medium roasted is 2,780. This value is for liquid 100 ml (3,38 ounces). This is a good source because you can easily drink 200ml of coffee in a day if you are a coffee drinker. One cup of coffee can have more antioxidants than the entire breakfast. Red wine will give a value of 3,607, green tea of 1,253 and cocoa powder is 55,653 for 100 grams. "Raw" cocoa powder can be as high as 80,000 units. If you want to drink a coffee, espresso is a better choice. Espresso will have 12,640 units on an ORAC scale but again this is for 100ml and you will drink one-third of that in a single espresso. When you start to read and understand some of the science behind antioxidants and you start to learn about ORAC values this could, and in most of the situations will impact your day to day grocery decisions. Most people don't want to die from cancer or have debilitating chronic diseases. You might, for example, substitute one food item for more nutritious one or god forbid you might decide to eat some nice fruit salad instead of the ice cream and Coca Cola. This is what made the industry so angry. As a consequence of this US government decided to quietly remove the ORAC database and to downplay all of the science behind it. Soon after it was published the USDA removed the database and the accepted line of "5 a Day" was adopted instead. Officially the ORAC database previously available on the USDA website has been withdrawn for the following two main reasons:

1. "ORAC values are routinely misused by food and dietary supplement manufacturing companies to promote their products and by consumers to guide their food and dietary supplement choices."

2. "The data for antioxidant capacity of foods generated by in vitro (test-tube) methods cannot be extrapolated to in vivo (human) effects and the clinical trials to test benefits of dietary antioxidants have produced mixed results. We know now that antioxidant molecules in food have a wide range of functions, many of which are unrelated to the ability to absorb free radicals."

There is a partial truth in some of the claims that USDA made but the decision was less motivated by science then desire to protect the interest of industry, both food and drug one. There is a truth that some food manufacturers started to label their products with health claims and that there is no science for every food item listed in the database but science is not the reason the database is withdrawn. It is correct that these in vitro measurements cannot be directly transported to in vivo subjects. There is an issue of bioavailability and potency. Phytochemicals from some food items can have a much higher ORAC rate in the test tube but poor absorbance so their real value is diminished and some other phytochemicals can be very potent but then cause other serious issues in the body. But again, at the end of the line, the database was still a very useful tool as a base for further research. USDA has gone so far to claim that antioxidants themselves are unproven to be beneficial for a human organism and by now you will understand that this is just another half-truth. One of the lies they keep repeating over and over again is: "ORAC values have been exaggerated and incorrectly linked to unsupported health claims." All of the science and citations I have in this chapter are well known and there are tens of thousands of studies by now and the science is here but only for the use in research for the new and improved patented medicine. Publicly available databases and awareness are not in the main interest of the US government. Unfortunately, most of us will have to educate ourselves and advice we will get will be designed to confuse us. My advice that I practice also in my life is to have at least 30,000 units a day from whole food sources. But I do not smoke and I exercise almost every day and eat mostly whole plant foods so I don't have a problem with consuming this amount. Also, I take some of the herbal mixtures that I make myself that will give me about 20,000 units in a tablespoon plus I do take some of the supplements like astaxanthin. I will consume 20 to 30 times the amount of accepted FDA recommended value. Most of the people, on the other hand, don't have an awareness of this issue. They know that they should eat fruit and vegetables because they are healthy but that is as far as awareness goes. And this is done deliberately. When I recommend something that is not in line with accepted FDA recommendations I do it on a base of accepted science and people usually have a hard time believing that FDA will do the opposite.

There was, for example, one study that did research into this exact topic (Food selection based on high total antioxidant capacity improves endothelial function in a low cardiovascular risk population. doi: 10.1016/j.numecd.2010.04.001). Researchers wanted to see the impact of a diet rich in antioxidants on endothelial function. They did a scientific study on dietary choices. Exactly what I discussed in this chapter and it is well-done study and people at the USDA should have read it before removing the ORAC database. They had two groups of people. Both have consumed a diet that has the same amount of fruit and vegetables. The difference was that one group had high quality produce rich in antioxidants like berries and the other group had a diet made out of poor quality choices like lettuce and cucumbers and bananas. The amount of fiber, protein, minerals, vitamins and all other nutrients were the same in both groups and were all above recommended RDA. The only difference was in the ORAC values of the diets. The result was as expected. The C-reactive protein (a marker for inflammation within the body) actually increased by 40 percent in the low antioxidant group compared to control and decreased 14 percent in a high antioxidant group. This can then be translated to all other diseases where chronic inflammation plays a role like cardiovascular disease. The conclusion was: "A short-term HT (antioxidant rich) diet improves endothelial function in volunteers at low cardiovascular risk, which may further reduce their risk of CVD (cardiovascular disease)." My recommendation will be to choose high antioxidant rich food choices if you can. If you want to eat salad eat kale instead of lettuce. If you want to eat fruit eat berries instead of bananas. If you want a beverage drink hibiscus tea instead of Coke. If you have some pro-inflammatory condition this will improve your health significantly. There are many diseases out there that are caused by inflammation that many people don't know that they are caused by a bad pro-inflammatory diet.

Depression is one of them (Inflamed moods: a review of the interactions between inflammation and mood disorders. doi: 10.1016/j.pnpbp.2014.01.013). For some people, it is bad genetics that plays a role, but for some, it is a bad diet and in both cases antioxidant-rich food will help. If you suffer from mood disorders disregard USDA recommendations and eat as many antioxidants as you can. "Accumulating evidence implicates inflammation as a critical mediator in the pathophysiology of mood disorders. Indeed, elevated levels of pro-inflammatory cytokines have been repeatedly demonstrated in both major depressive disorder (MDD) and bipolar disorder (BD) patients. Further, the induction of a pro-inflammatory state in healthy or medically ill subjects induces 'sickness behavior' resembling depressive symptomatology. Potential mechanisms involved include, but are not limited to, direct effects of pro-inflammatory cytokines on monoamine levels, dysregulation of the hypothalamic-pituitary-adrenal (HPA) axis, pathologic microglial cell activation, impaired neuroplasticity and structural and functional brain changes. Anti-inflammatory agents, such as acetyl-salicylic acid (ASA), celecoxib, anti-TNF-α agents, minocycline, curcumin and omega-3 fatty acids, are being investigated for use in mood disorders. Current evidence shows improved outcomes in mood disorder patients when anti-inflammatory agents are used as an adjunct to conventional therapy." This makes sense if we understand how evolution works. If depression does not have an evolutionary protective role for the species it will be selected against. The high rate of mood disorders in our current society is a consequence of adaptive benefit. The problem is a shift in environment and diet. The theory goes that depression is an evolutionary strategy for infection control. If you have a virus that is life-threatening you will be put into isolation to prevent the spread of infection. Depression does the same thing. In the stone age for example infection was a leading cause of death and more than half of the children died before reaching puberty. Life expectancy was 25 years of age. The theory was made that if one individual gets influenza or some other life-threatening disease the instinct of that individual will be to become irritated, depressed and antisocial on top of all of the visible signs of sickness. It is not the pain that causes depression but overall inflammation. This is bad for individual but if we look at the overall survival of the species it is beneficial (Depression as an evolutionary strategy for defense against infection. doi: 10.1016/j.bbi.2012.12.002). Individuals that have some sort of health issues and that have inflammation no matter what source of that inflammation might be, will as a theory goes suffer from the additional shift in brain chemistry. That will make them depressed, irritable and angry as an instinctive underlying mechanism. The purpose is to isolate that individual until the infection is gone so that the spread of infection is minimized. But what happens if the source of that infection is not some life-threatening virus but a bad and pro-inflammatory diet? There are animal species like honey bees that will leave to die alone if they are sick. This is not something new. This connection was well known for almost a hundred years now. If doctors give people drugs that induce inflammation the depression will be induced as well. More than 50 percent of people that receive interferon develop severe forms of clinical depression. Lacking an adequate level of antioxidants in a diet plus the addition of all environmental toxins and plus dead meat bacteria endotoxins will be pro-inflammatory and depression inducing. Endotoxins are part of the outer membrane of the cell wall of gram-negative bacteria. They are released from bacteria when they die, their cell walls get destroyed and cannot be cooked away any further. There is a lot of dead bacteria in meat and this is one of the reasons why meat is so pro-inflammatory on top of other factors. We can cook the meat but endotoxins will remain. In experiments done in vivo after injecting endotoxins directly into human subjects, the autoimmune reaction and inflammation were significant and have led to significant increases (from baseline) in IL-6 and TNF-alpha levels as well as feelings of social disconnection and depressed mood (Inflammation and social experience: an inflammatory challenge induces feelings of social disconnection in addition to depressed mood doi: 10.1016/j.bbi.2009.12.009). Also, there were other experiments that proved this by brain imaging. In people injected with endotoxins brain imaging showed a lack of normal excitement to pleasurable stimulation known as anhedonia (Inflammation-induced anhedonia: endotoxin reduces ventral striatum responses to reward. doi: 10.1016/j.biopsych.2010.06.010). Inflammation changes reward-related neural responding in humans forcing us to become nonresponsive to pleasurable stimulation where we will need stronger stimuli to exert the same effects and then this can create pleasure seeking behavior, binge eating, and depressed mood. My recommendation to patients that have any type of mood disorder is to try to remove pro-inflammatory foods from their diet and that includes all animal products plus a wide range of other vegan products as well and then to dramatically increase the ORAC units score of their diet.

One other medical condition that I want to mention where it has been proven that a high antioxidant diet can help and prevent is periodontal disease. And this means much more than just 3000 to 5000 units that USDA recommends. In nature, there is no toothbrush or any form of dental hygiene. If we look at our primate cousins in wilderness periodontal disease is rare and they do not brush their teeth. If we look at the skeletal remains from people that lived in the stone age period there are skulls with perfect teeth. It is correct that sugar is the main reason we have an epidemic of dental disease these days but it is not the only one. When you stop brushing your teeth, the plaque starts to build up and eventually the gums will get inflamed. In time the infection will go deeper into the gums to the supporting structure of the tooth causing periodontal disease. There was an experiment where subjects had to stop brushing and they had plaque buildup but also in the experiment they were eating paleo type diet. The result was that although the plaque did build up their inflammation of the gums actually decreased (The impact of the stone age diet on gingival conditions in the absence of oral hygiene. doi: 10.1902/jop.2009.080376). The combination of the absence of sugar as a food source for bad bacteria that live in our mouth plus an increase in anti-inflammatory foods rich in phytochemicals has led to a significant decrease in the number of bacteria that were present. In the line of other experiments, it was shown that lycopene, for example, has anti-bacterial and anti-inflammatory properties and that it helps when dealing with gingivitis.

At the end, if you do accept the standard line of accepted ideology that was pushed by USDA and decide that antioxidant-rich diet is not of significant value to overall health because body can only utilize 3000 to 5000 ORAC units a day and that the rest of it is just going to waste then you will also have to accept the officially recognized line that if you do consume more antioxidants in a whole food way they will do you no harm either. In this chapter, I have listed a number of diseases that do benefit from an increase in antioxidant consumption. So how can we increase our antioxidant score? Well, we will have to do the analysis of the total antioxidant content of more than 3100 foods in already mention study to see how to optimize our diet. I am going to use some quotes from the study and then I will analyze some of the most potent and antioxidant rich foods in the chart and then we can see what is the most optimal and easiest way to increase the antioxidant content of our diet.

"A plant-based diet protects against chronic oxidative stress-related diseases... It is widely accepted that a plant-based diet with a high intake of fruits, vegetables, and other nutrient-rich plant foods may reduce the risk of oxidative stress-related diseases... Spices, herbs, and supplements include the most antioxidant-rich products in our study, some exceptionally high. Berries, fruits, nuts, chocolate, vegetables, and products thereof constitute common foods and beverages with high antioxidant values... Plant-based foods introduce significantly more antioxidants into the human diet than non-plant foods... Most bioactive food constituents are derived from plants; those so derived are collectively called phytochemicals. The large majority of these phytochemicals are redox-active molecules and therefore defined as anti-oxidants. Antioxidants can eliminate free radicals and other reactive oxygen and nitrogen species, and these reactive species contribute to most chronic diseases. It is hypothesized that antioxidants originating from foods may work as antioxidants in their own right in vivo, as well as bring about beneficial health effects through other mechanisms, including acting as inducers of mechanisms related to antioxidant defense, longevity, cell maintenance, and DNA repair... There is not necessarily a direct relationship between the antioxidant content of a food sample consumed and the subsequent antioxidant activity in the target cell. Factors influencing the bioavailability of phytochemical antioxidants include the food matrix, absorption, and metabolism."

"The highest antioxidant values in the beverages category were found among the unprocessed tea leaves, tea powders, and coffee beans... Other antioxidant rich beverages are red wine, which have a smaller variation of antioxidant content (1.78 to 3.66 mmol/100 g), pomegranate juice, prepared green tea (0.57 to 2.62 mmol/100 g), grape juice, prune juice and black tea (0.75 to 1.21 mmol/100 g). Beer, soft drinks and ginger ale contain the least antioxidants of the beverages in our study, with drinking water completely devoid of antioxidants..."

The values that are given here are in mmol/100g and 1 mmol is 1000 micromole ORAC units. For example, 3.66 mmol/100 g is 3660 ORAC units.

"The dairy category included 86 products and the majority of these products were low in antioxidant content, in the range of 0.0 to 0.8 mmol/100 g. Eggs are almost devoid of antioxidants with the highest antioxidant values found in egg yolk (0.16 mmol/100 g)... When classifying the samples into the three main classes the difference in antioxidant content between plant- and animal-based foods become apparent. The results here uncover that the antioxidant content of foods varies several thousand-fold and that antioxidant rich foods originate from the plant kingdom while meat, fish and other foods from the animal kingdom are low in antioxidants. Comparing the mean value of the 'Meat and meat products' category with plant based categories, fruits, nuts, chocolate and berries have from 5 to 33 times higher mean antioxidant content than the mean of meat products. Diets comprised mainly of animal-based foods are thus low in antioxidant content while diets based mainly on a variety of plant-based foods are antioxidant rich, due to the thousands of bioactive antioxidant phytochemicals found in plants which are conserved in many foods and beverages... Nuts are a rich source of many important nutrients and some are also antioxidant-rich... Most of the spices and herbs analyzed have particularly high antioxidant contents. Although spices and herbs contribute little weight on the dinner plate, they may still be important contributors to our antioxidant intake, especially in dietary cultures where spices and herbs are used regularly. We interpret the elevated concentration of antioxidants observed in several dried herbs compared to fresh samples, as a normal consequence of the drying process leaving most of the antioxidants intact in the dried end product. This tendency is also seen in some fruits and their dried counterparts. Thus, dried herbs and fruit are potentially excellent sources of antioxidants... Herbal and traditional plant medicines emerged as many of the highest antioxidant-containing products in our study. We speculate that the high inherent antioxidant property of many plants is an important contributor to the herb's medicinal qualities... With their high content of phytochemicals such as flavonoids, tannins, stilbenoids, phenolic acids, and lignans berries and berry products are potentially excellent antioxidant sources... During the processing of berries to jams, total phenol content is reduced resulting in lower antioxidant values in processed berry products than in fresh berries... Differences in unprocessed and processed plant food samples are also seen in our study where processed berry products like jam and syrup have approximately half the antioxidant capacity of fresh berries. On the other hand, processing may also enhance a food's potential by increasing the number of antioxidants released from the food matrix, which otherwise would be less or not at all available for absorption. Processing of tomato is one such example where lycopene from heat-processed tomato sauce is more bioavailable than unprocessed tomato... It is not likely that all antioxidant-rich foods are good sources and that all antioxidants provided in the diet are bioactive. Bioavailability differs greatly from one phytochemical to another, so the most antioxidant rich foods in our diet are not necessarily those leading to the highest concentrations of active metabolites in target tissues… Biochemically active phytochemicals found in plant-based foods also have many powerful biological properties which are not necessarily correlated with their antioxidant capacity, including acting as inducers of antioxidant defense mechanisms in vivo or as gene expression modulators. Thus, a food low in antioxidant content may have beneficial health effects due to other food components or phytochemicals executing bioactivity through other mechanisms."

This is one of those studies that have the potential to revolutionize a nutritional science but not only that. This study has practical and real implications on our day to day grocery decisions. The sad reality is that the vast majority of people don't want to eat healthy and don't want to learn and don't want to do anything that they don't need to do. Only when there is a chronic condition there is essentially an incentive for diet optimization for most of the people. Because of this, I will try to give some easy to do and cost-effective ways to increase the antioxidant intake. For most of the people, cheap and easy solutions will be the only ones that they will follow. If you want to go one step further than you can try to completely optimize your diet. The first and easiest step to do is to analyze the most antioxidant rich food list and then just add them to your diet without changing anything. This is the same way as taking a multivitamin once a day. If you don't want to give up meat, and sugar, and fat, and alcohol, and smoking you can try at least to add a tablespoon of turmeric a day, or a cup of cocoa, or hibiscus tea in a day. There are foods that are so antioxidant rich that essentially we can take them as a supplement without even thinking about our diet and just this act will have an impact on our health. Let's take a look at the list of the first 25 of the most antioxidant rich foods that were given by now removed USDA database.

FOOD ITEM		ORAC Value (μmol TE/100 g)
1.	Dragon's Blood (Sangre de Grado) (Croton lechleri)	2,897,110
2.	Clove, essential oil	1,078,700
3.	Triphala Powder	706,250
4.	Catechin 100, Green-tea capsules, extract	536,050
5.	Coffee Cherry (Cascara) Powder	343,900
6.	Sumac Bran, Raw	312,400
7.	Ground Cloves	290,283
8.	Indian Gooseberry (Amla Berries), Dried	261,530
9.	Sorghum Bran, Raw	240,000
10.	Rosemary Spice, Dried	165,280
11.	Meadowsweet (Filipendula ulmaria), flower, dried	167,820
12.	Tea, instant, dry powder	165,860
13.	Peppermint Leaves, Dried	160,820
14.	Thyme Spice, Dried	157,380
15.	Chaga Mushroom Extract	146,700
16.	Baobab Fruit Powder, Dried	140,000
17.	Wild marjoram, leaves, dried	131,920
18.	Cinnamon Spice, Ground	131,420
19.	Turmeric Spice, Ground	127,680
20.	Black Cohosh Root, Dried	126,495
21.	Lemon balm, leaves, dried	125,330
22.	Vanilla Bean Spice, Dried	122,400
23.	Sage Spice, Ground	119,929

| 24. | Grape Seed Extract | 108,130 |
| 25. | Acai, fruit pulp/skin, powder | 102,700 |

Besides the first 25 that I listed here as an example there are food items that also have good antioxidant potential for everyday use even if they are not as potent. There are also some food items that might seem like a rich source of antioxidants but actually, they are not.

• Allspice, Ground	100,400
• Oregano Spice, Dried	89,510
• Parsley Spice, Dried	73,670
• Basil Spice, Dried	61,063
• Cocoa Powder, Unsweetened	55,653
• Curry Spices Powder	48,504
• Ginger Spice, Ground	39,041
• Black Pepper Spice	34,053
• Barberries, Dried	27,300
• Pecans, with a pellicle, Raw	17,940
• English Walnuts, Raw	13,541
• Prunes (Dried Plums)	8,059
• Pinto Beans, Raw	8,033
• Black Currants (European), Raw	7,957
• Pistachio Nuts, Raw	7,675
• Sunflower seeds, Raw	7,500
• White Chia Seeds, Raw	7,000
• Hibiscus Tea, Brewed	6,990
• Plums, Raw	6,100
• Blueberries, Raw	4,669

- Artichokes, Boiled — 4,540
- Strawberries, Raw — 4,302
- Red Delicious Apples With Skin, Raw — 4,275
- Curly kale, Red — 4,090
- Deglet Noor Dates — 3,895
- Sweet Cherries, Raw — 3,747
- Peanut butter, smooth style — 3,432
- Raisins, Seedless — 3,406
- Red Cabbage (Purple), Boiled — 3,145
- Brewed Arabica Coffee, Medium Roast — 2,780
- Red Cabbage (Purple), Raw — 2,496
- Concord Grape Juice — 2,389
- Broccoli, Boiled — 2,160
- Sweet Potato, Baked In Skin — 2,115
- Oranges, All Varieties, Raw — 2,103
- Cashew nuts, Raw — 1,948
- Green Kale, Raw — 1,770
- Black Grapes, Raw — 1,746
- Macadamia nuts, Dry Roasted — 1,695
- Frozen Spinach (Chopped or Leaf), Unprepared — 1,687
- Pistachios, roasted — 1,380
- Lemons Without Peel, Raw — 1,346
- Green Tea, Brewed — 1,253
- Sesame seeds, Raw — 1,210
- Potatoes, white, flesh and skin, baked — 1,138
- Ground Flaxseed, Raw — 1,130
- Pinto Beans, Boiled — 904

- Paste, canned tomato   880
- Kiwi Fruit, Raw   862
- Red Peppers, Raw   821
- Bananas, Raw   795
- Orange Juice, Raw   726
- Carrots, Raw   697
- White Button Mushrooms   691
- Cabbage, Raw   529
- Iceberg Lettuce   438
- Green Beans, Canned   290
- Brown Rice, Basmati, Cooked   270
- Honey   130
- Canned Green Peas   120
- Limes, Raw   82
- Milk, 1% Fat   50
- Egg Yolk   20

The whole list of all ORAC values can be found in the study that I had referenced but not on the USDA website anymore. I have just used some examples here. When you learn the basics if you want you can always hire a professional nutritionist or learn more by yourself. Consider this chapter as a starting point. Also, all of the values listed here are just approximations, an average value from a range of different values and are not to be taken on face value. The ORAC values listed here are meant for us to have an insight into the potency of some food items. For instance, value for ground cloves has a range from 125,550 units measured in a sample obtained from the USA to a value of 465,320 for a sample obtained from Black Boy, Rieber og søn, Norway. The average would be around 290,000. The ground cinnamon, for example, has values that range from 17,650 to 139,890. Most of the values listed here, or on other sources are again in a practical sense exaggerated. The antioxidant value starts to drop immediately after the produce is removed from the field. The longer it sits on a shelf the lower the antioxidant value will be. Also, if food is exposed to the air it will eventually go rancid. Nuts and seeds have a shell that protects them from oxygen but if the shell is broken then the oxidation can accrue. That is the reason why it is never a good idea to buy already grounded nuts or seeds. If you want flaxseed, sesame seed or any other seed buy them whole and grind them yourself before consumption. If you want to use fresh fruits or vegetables to make a smoothie if you don't have vacuum blender there is a good possibility that you will diminish most of the antioxidants in them. It is always a better choice to eat whole fruit than to blend them but there are recipes that demand the use of powerful blenders so keep this in mind or find a vacuum blender. If you want to juice then use masticating juicers. They use pressure and low RPMs to squeeze out the juice without blending it at high speed. This will help to lower the oxidation and the juice will have a better taste and color. The use of masticating juicers is an excellent way for everyone to increase the nutritional density of their diet because it is simulating the process of digestion by removing the fiber out. When you remove the fiber then the rest of the juice can be digested with no problem in a very short period. If you don't eat enough fiber then this can be a problem but if you do have adequate fiber intake then juicing high quality, nutritious, low-calorie vegetables will infuse you with a lot of micronutrients without increasing the caloric intake during the day. Juicing high-quality low-calorie vegetables with a lot of antioxidants and minerals is unnatural practice, but in a positive way. In nature, we would not be able to consume a large number of high fiber vegetables but if we remove the fiber and only drink the juice, there is no issue. Keep this in mind, every grinding or blending or any exposure to the air will reduce the antioxidant value of the produce. If you want cloves, buy them whole and grind them yourself before use.

When you look at the values in the chart you can see that in most of the cases dried fruit will have more antioxidants than fresh produce and this is just an illusion. Because most of the fruit is water if we remove that water the rest of the fruit will become lighter and will have more fruit for the same 100 grams. Micronutrient density of the dried fruit, vegetables and spices can only be the same or worse. Because the sugar is not evaporated the number of micronutrients per one calorie remains the same as in the fresh produce. The only difference is that now it is more concentrated produce because the water has evaporated so we can have an illusion that somehow the dried rosemary is better than the fresh one. It is on a gram to gram bases but it is not on a calorie to calorie basis. On an antioxidant value chart, it is always the case that we can see that fresh herb or fruit has a lower ORAC value than the dried ones. Also, the dried ones will always have a lower score than the extract or an extracted oil. That is why we can see for instance that grounded cloves have an antioxidant capacity of 290,000 and the extracted clove oil has more than one million. Or for instance, fresh green tea leaves will have lower ORAC value than the dried ones and the dried ones will have a lower value than the green tea extract in a pill. There is a list of more than

100 different essential oils but I did not include them in the chart. I included only the clove oil that is the most powerful of them all. I didn't include the values because they are higher than any other produce in the list. Essential oils will have taken more than 20 of 25 most potent antioxidant-rich foods in existence because in an essence they are concentrated forms of phytochemicals.

The golden rule is something like this. Most powerful antioxidants are a concentrated form of natural antioxidant rich herbs. On top of the list will be essential oils, herbal extracts, dried herbs, and powders. Then we will have dried fruit, and superfoods like antioxidant-rich fruit, raw nuts, and seeds and vegetables. Then there will be regular fruit, regular vegetables, and then at the very end will be a whole list of animal products that have no antioxidant value and are actually pro-inflammatory. In essence, all animal products have negative ORAC values if we understand what in the reality they do in our bodies. Also, you can see in the chart that in most cases heat destroys some of the ORAC value. Row beans and nuts are good examples. Raw pinto beans have a score of 8,033 and raw pistachio nuts of 7,675. Boiled pinto beans will have a score of only 904 and roasted pistachios of 1,380. It is the same story with green beans, green peas and most of the other beans and seeds and nuts and most of the fruit and vegetables but again not all of them. There are exceptions. For example, raw sweet potato will have an ORAC value of 902 but baked sweet potato will have a score of 2115. Raw red cabbage will have a score of 2496 but boiled red cabbage will have 3145. This is because of the bioavailability of the antioxidants. In some cases, heat destroys the cells and allows the phytochemicals to leech out. It is the same with tomatoes because of the lycopene. Also, some of the water content is evaporated creating a more concentrated source of antioxidants. "How to cook the broccoli" was always the question but in reality, the ORAC value actually increases by about 33% after boiling. Unlike most veggies, the types of antioxidants in broccoli are not greatly affected by the heat of cooking except for the sulforaphane. Sulforaphane is the reason you will want to eat cruciferous vegetables in the first place. It is a phytochemical that is unique in cruciferous vegetables family and antioxidants you can find in other foods. It is derived nearly exclusively from cruciferous vegetables. You could eat as much as you want of other kinds of vegetables there will be no sulforaphane in there if you didn't eat something cruciferous. I already wrote about the "hack and hold" tactic that we can use to increase the sulforaphane concentrations in the first book so I won't do it again but it is unique and very potent phytochemical especially for phase 2 detoxification process. If you buy frozen broccoli or kale the myrosinase enzyme is destroyed and there will be no sulforaphane creation and that is the reason why fresh kale fights cancer ten times as much as frozen. The freezing process is generally regarded as destructive to antioxidant capacity compared to fresh produce. When we look at these items we have to take into consideration not just the overall antioxidant potency, but how many calories will come with those antioxidants. The most important issue of them all is how much, in reality, will we be able to consume some food item. For instance, cabbage is not an antioxidant star but it has very little calories so when we consider the number of ORAC units per calorie it is actually a good source. But then again cabbage is hard to eat in large quantities and herbs and spices have that convenience that they can add a significant antioxidant power in a single pinch. In the end, we will have to analyze individual foods and groups of the foods to form some of the nutrition rules.

First on the list, and so far the most potent source of antioxidants with a value greater than 2 million is already mentioned Sangre de grado. When the trunk of the Croton lechleri tree is cut or wounded, a dark red, sappy resin oozes out that is one of the world's most powerful antioxidant. It has a long history of indigenous use in the rainforest of South America. The earliest written reference dates its use to the 1600s when Spanish naturalist and explorer P. Bernabé Cobo found that the curative power of the sap was widely known throughout the indigenous tribes of Mexico, Peru, and Ecuador. In Brazilian traditional medicine, the sap is used for wounds, hemorrhaging, diarrhea, mouth ulcers, and as a general tonic. In modern times, it is considered an antioxidant dietary supplement but it has one big problem. A study from 2003 found it had mutagenic activity when tested against Salmonella typhimurium strains (Evaluation of the mutagenic, antimutagenic and antiproliferative potential of Croton lechleri (Muell. Arg.) latex. Phytomedicine. 2003 Mar;10(2-3):139-44). One year later another study found mutagenic activity when it was tested against two Salmonella typhimurium strains. It took almost a decade until 2013 when another paper was published on this topic. Rather than finding it to be a mutagen, they founded the opposite, that it was a "possible mutagen-protective food ingredient" (Croton lechleri Müll. Arg. (Euphorbiaceae) stem bark essential oil as possible mutagen-protective food ingredient against heterocyclic amines from cooked food. doi: 10.1016/j.foodchem.2013.01.076). Now because of the conflicting science maybe it will be the best option to avoid this supplement until more research is done.

Number two on the list is clove essential oil. It is the most potent of essential oils and also at the same time the most popular of them all. It is so popular that we can find this oil almost at every health food store or pharmacy. People like this oil not because it is one of the most antioxidant-rich substances in existence but because it has a very nice aroma. It is sweet as vanilla and spicy as pepper at the same time. It has the best scent according to most consumers. The main active component responsible for the smell – eugenol (acetyl eugenol) – is so strong that just a couple drops in a diffuser will engulf a small room with this sweet peppery aroma. It is so potent because the cloves themselves are one of the most potent herbs with an ORAC value of 290,283 so it should not come as a surprise that oil extract will be four-times as powerful. Even among essential oils, it is a superstar. Second on the essential oil list on the ORAC potency is myrrh essential oil with a 65% lower value. Clove essential oil is extremely powerful and concentrated and should never be taken in undiluted form. If it touches the skin it can cause irritation. If you try to consume this oil it will cause damage to gums and dental tissue and will burn your mouth and throat. When it reaches the stomach, it can cause abdominal pain, diarrhea, and vomiting. Also, it has very potent anticoagulant/antiplatelet activity in the bloodstream and can cause increased bleeding due to less blood clotting. One of the myths you will hear is that clove oil kills nerves. That's not how its numbing mechanism works. Before a Lidocaine or Novocain injection, dentists use to swab your gums with it for 5 minutes for some preliminary anesthetic action (today they use more effective chemicals). The eugenol works like other local anesthetics, by temporarily blocking the nerves that carry the pain signal to your brain. There is no "killing" of the nerves involved, as some people believe. Today there are a number of studies that have found a range of different benefits of cloves both in terms of ground cloves and as on oil. They work and are the same in a sense. In this study from 2012 (Antimicrobial Effect of Clove and Lemongrass Oils against Planktonic Cells and Biofilms of Staphylococcus aureus. S. Chamdit and P. Siripermpool) researchers have found that clove oil had the ability to kill staph bacteria cells in liquid culture and in biofilm. A biofilm is a community of bacteria that lives together, shielded by a protective slimy film. Most antibiotics aren't effective at penetrating the biofilm and killing staph bacteria but according to this study, clove oil seems to be able to. A 2017 study (Antifungal activity of essential oils against fungi isolated from air. doi: 10.1080/10773525.2018.1447320) looked at the antifungal activity of several essential oils. Of the oils tested, clove oil was the most effective at stopping the growth of a range of fungi with environmental origins. Traditionally cloves have been used to fight inflamed gums both as an antibiotic and as a pain reliever. Today we can look at the cloves and clove oil as one of the most potent sources of antioxidants. Adding cloves to our diet will reap a line of benefits especially in people that already have nutrition and antioxidant depleted diets.

If you don't like the strong taste of cloves you can go to number three on the list, the Triphala Powder. It is one of the oldest and strongest Ayurvedic medicine. In Sanskrit, tri phala means three fruits and it is a powder that is made by mixing Indian gooseberry (Emblica officinalis), black myrobalan (Terminalia chebula) and belleric myrobalan (Terminalia bellirica). You can find this in almost any Indian store and it is relatively cheap. In studies, most of the benefits were correlated to its antioxidant capacity and this can be one of those supplements that can add tremendous amounts of antioxidants in a single pinch but there is a catch. One in five Ayurvedic herbal dietary supplements was found to be contaminated with lead, mercury or arsenic (Detection of toxic heavy metals and pesticide residue in herbal plants which are commonly used in the herbal formulations. doi: 10.1007/s10661-010-1828-2). There were cases of heavy metal poisoning for decades associated with ayurvedic medicine and it was a well-known fact even before the studies have been done. In many cases, people suffering from ayurvedic lead poisoning have higher lead concentrations than people suffering from paint removal poisoning. The good thing now is that we know what Ayurvedic medicine is toxic and which one is not. In the case of Triphala powder the levels of heavy metals including arsenic, mercury and lead exceed the recommended daily allowance (Lead, mercury, and arsenic in US- and Indian-manufactured Ayurvedic medicines sold via the Internet. doi: 10.1001/jama.300.8.915). There is no safe limit for heavy nerve toxins like mercury but again to have some perspective one serving of Triphala has 46 micrograms of mercury while one serving of white can tuna has 1345. But again, there are other completely clean and rich sources of antioxidants so there is no real necessity to consume Triphala. If you want rich antioxidant source you can go with Amla that is already in Triphala and unlike Triphala is completely clean.

Amla is a dried Indian gooseberry powder. It has an ORAC score of 261,530 and it is as potent as cloves. There is a lot of research actually done on amla and it has been found to be very effective against many diseases. Amla enjoys a mythical reputation in India due to a belief that it originated from drops of Amrit, the nectar of immortality. The Indian gooseberry tree is also supposed to have been used to achieve enlightenment by Phussa Buddha, the first Buddha of antiquity. In scientific research, it did prolong the lifespan of fruit flies and also increase their sexual behavior (The effect of Emblica officinalis diet on lifespan, sexual behavior, and fitness characters in Drosophila melanogaster. doi: 10.4103/0974-8520.92544). Also flies on amla laid more eggs and more eggs hatched as well. It did increase fertility and longevity so the ayurvedic tradition of immortality and its aphrodisiac effect properties might have been based on some traditional first-hand experience. If we look at real clinical studies done on humans, we will see the same benefits as with all other types of potent antioxidants. In this study (Effect of Amla fruit (Emblica officinalis Gaertn.) on blood glucose and lipid profile of normal subjects and type 2 diabetic patients. doi: 10.3109/09637486.2011.560565) just adding amla made a significant improvement in cholesterol both total and cholesterol profile. How much significance? One gooseberry a day cuts bad cholesterol and triglycerides in half in three weeks. In this study (A comparative clinical study of hypolipidemic efficacy of Amla (Emblica officinalis) with 3-hydroxy-3-methylglutaryl-coenzyme-A reductase inhibitor simvastatin. doi: 10.4103/0253-7613.93857) they compared the effect of amla on lowering cholesterol with leading cholesterol-lowering drug simvastatin known as a Zocor. It lowered total cholesterol the same as Zocor to around 15 percent but there is one problem with this study. They only used 500mg of amla. That is half of one gram and they didn't even use dried power of amla but dried fruit juice powder of amla. But even this pinch of amla juice powder provided the same effects as a statin. If you want a new cholesterol-lowering drug, well here is a new one called amla that probably won't be mention to you by your cardiologist at all. No prescription needed and it costs 5 cents a dose. Plus, you will get all other benefits from it as a side effect. It will also reduce arterial stiffness and overall inflammation in the body. Amla also has around 60 percent the potency of blood-thinning effect as aspirin or Plavix (Study of pharmacodynamic interaction of Phyllanthus emblica extract with clopidogrel and ecosprin in patients with type II diabetes mellitus. doi: 10.1016/j.phymed.2013.10.024). If you have any type of cardiovascular disease this will be one of the supplements you will be smart to incorporate into a daily routine. Also, the study above that I referenced is actually a study on the effects of amla on type 2 diabetes. Amla was outperforming leading diabetic drug glyburide sold as Diabeta. One-quarter of a teaspoon of amla is as potent at fighting type 2 diabetes as billions of dollars' worth of research pharmaceutical patented medicine. One of the side effects of Diabeta is liver failure or poisoning of bone merrow. It is also considered as a very potent chemotherapy agent in fighting cancer (Amla (Emblica officinalis Gaertn), a wonder berry in the treatment and prevention of cancer. doi: 10.1097/CEJ.0b013e32834473f4). Here is a brief summary of this study: "The fruit is used either alone or in combination with other plants to treat many ailments such as common cold and fever; as a diuretic, laxative, liver tonic, refrigerant, stomachic, restorative, alterative, antipyretic, anti-inflammatory, hair tonic; to prevent peptic ulcer and dyspepsia, and as a digestive. Preclinical studies have shown that amla possesses antipyretic, analgesic, antitussive, antiatherogenic, adaptogenic, cardioprotective, gastroprotective, antianemia, antihypercholesterolemia, wound healing, antidiarrheal, antiatherosclerotic, hepatoprotective, nephroprotective, and neuroprotective properties. In addition, experimental studies have shown that amla and some of its phytochemicals such as gallic acid, ellagic acid, pyrogallol, some norsesquiterpenoids, corilagin, geraniin, elaeocarpusin, and prodelphinidins B1 and B2 also possess antineoplastic effects. Amla is also reported to possess radiomodulatory, chemomodulatory, chemopreventive effects, free radical scavenging, antioxidant, anti-inflammatory, antimutagenic and immunomodulatory activities, properties that are efficacious in the treatment and prevention of cancer." It basically helps with everything ever tested. If you have a condition no matter what it is it is a great possibility that amla can help. It is even used as a snake venom neutralizing agent. And to top it all, it kills cancer cells with such potency that will rival most of the strongest chemotherapy drugs currently used in cancer treatment. Unlike chemotherapy, you can take amla year-round for the rest of your life. It is considered to be the wonder drug in alternative medicine when dealing with cancer prevention and treatment. It is so potent that Big

Pharma refuses to research this berry. There is only sporadic research done from more independent sources. In this study (Antitumour effects of Phyllanthus emblica L.: induction of cancer cell apoptosis and inhibition of in vivo tumour promotion and in vitro invasion of human cancer cells. doi: 10.1002/ptr.3127) they tested amla against six different types of human cancers. The result was that amla decreased cancer cell growth and then as a concentration increased it actually completely stopped the growth of all six cancers. As a concentration was raised the cancer growth became negative and cancer cells began to die off and eventually when the experiment was stopped there was a reduction of more than 60 percent in size of all six types of cancers. It destroyed cancer so profoundly that it was remarkable. The best thing about it all is that at the highest concentration of amla that killed off more than 60 percent of cancer cells it didn't have an impact on normal cells. This study defined amla as one of the strongest chemotherapy agents so far because of this one simple reason. Amla can be taken in high dosages year-round with no negative side effects what so ever. Only positive health effects are side effects of amla.

On a fourth place on the list is green tea extract. Green tea is used as a traditional Indian and Chinese medicine and today in modern time there is a long line of research of all of its benefits. People who take green tea extract in a supplemental form usually do this because of the effects that green tea has on the body. It is not viewed necessarily as an antioxidant supplement but it could be viewed also as a good source of antioxidants independently from all of its unique health effects. Tea is the most consumed beverage in the world behind water. However, 78 percent of the tea consumed worldwide is black and only about 20 percent is green. All types of tea, except herbal tea, are brewed from the dried leaves of the Camellia sinensis bush. The level of oxidation of the leaves determines the type of tea. Green tea is made from unoxidized leaves and is one of the less processed types of tea. It, therefore, contains the most antioxidants and beneficial polyphenols. Because of its antioxidant properties, modern studies have shown that it has the healing abilities in fighting all of the diseases where antioxidants usually help plus everything from weight loss to Alzheimer's disease to anxiety. One unique chemical that is present in a larger concentration in green tea is Epigallocatechin gallate (EGCG). EGCG in green tea may offer a variety of health benefits, such as reduced inflammation, weight loss, and the prevention of heart and brain diseases. In studies, it has proven benefits in cancer prevention and also in boosting immune antiviral function. Women who drank most of the green tea had a 20-30% lower risk of developing breast cancer (Green tea consumption and breast cancer risk or recurrence: a meta-analysis. doi: 10.1007/s10549-009-0415-0). Men who drink green tea had a 48% lower risk of developing prostate cancer (Green tea consumption and prostate cancer risk in Japanese men: a prospective study. Am J Epidemiol. 2008 Jan 1;167(1):71-7). People who drink green tea were up to 42% less likely to develop colorectal cancer (An inverse association between tea consumption and colorectal cancer risk. doi: 10.18632/oncotarget.16959). Most people are aware of the anti-cancer abilities of green tea but what is not so common knowledge is that green tea is one of the best immune system boosters that exists and it is not the consequence of its antioxidant power. Dating back to the military medical journal of 1906 it was a practice that servicemen fill their canteens with tea to kill off the bugs that cause typhoid fever.

Then back in the 1990s, there was a new line of studies that looked into the antiviral properties of green tea. It was discovered that external genital warts resulting from the human papillomavirus can be healed completely in more than 50 percent of cases without heavy synthetic drugs by just using green tea ointment (Sinecatechins 10% ointment: a green tea extract for the treatment of external genital warts. Skin Therapy Lett. 2015 Jan-Feb;20(1):6-8). This might not be a life-threatening virus but for some people, common influenza can be fatal. Elderly people have a high immunity boost from drinking green tea and in some cases, it might even prevent them from developing life-threatening influenza. Health workers that drink green tea come down with the flu three times less often (Effects of green tea catechins and theanine on preventing influenza infection among healthcare workers: a randomized controlled trial. doi: 10.1186/1472-6882-11-15). Even just gargling with a green tea can prevent influenza in elderly nursing homes by 8-fold (Gargling with tea catechin extracts for the prevention of influenza infection in elderly nursing home residents: a prospective clinical study. J Altern Complement Med. 2006 Sep;12(7):669-72). This is a unique health boosting effect of green tea on top of its antioxidant power. The way that green tea boosts the immune system is by increasing cell division and activity of gamma, delta T cells (Specific formulation of Camellia sinensis prevents cold and flu symptoms and enhances gamma, delta T cell function: a randomized, double-blind, placebo-controlled study. J Am Coll Nutr. 2007 Oct;26(5):445-52). If you drink six cups of green tea a day there will be a 15-fold increase in interferon-gamma production in a time period as short as one week. That is a large increase. Why this happens is a complicated science, if you want you can read it more in this study (Antigens in tea-beverage prime human Vgamma 2Vdelta 2 T cells in vitro and in vivo for memory and nonmemory antibacterial cytokine responses. Proc Natl Acad Sci U S A. 2003 May 13;100(10):6009-14. Epub 2003 Apr 28). "Human gammadelta T cells mediate innate immunity to microbes via T cell receptor-dependent recognition of unprocessed antigens. These nonpeptide alkylamine antigens are shared by tumor cells, bacteria, parasites, and fungi but also by edible plant products such as tea, apples, mushrooms, and wine. Priming of gammadelta T cells with alkylamine antigens in vitro results in a memory response to these antigens. Drinking tea, which contains l-theanine, a precursor of the nonpeptide antigen ethylamine, primed peripheral blood gammadelta T cells to mediate a memory response on reexposure to ethylamine and to secrete IFN-gamma in response to bacteria."

Why this is unique to tea is because of l-theanine. It is an amino acid that got its name from tea as theanine and it can be found only in two species in the entire ecosystem of the world. In tea and in one species of mushroom called Bay Bolete. It is because of l-theanine in the first place that green tea and tea, in general, is the most consumed beverage in the world. It is an amino acid that can cross the blood brain barrier and when it reaches the brain it has mood-altering effects. Tea also contains caffeine as well. Not in the same dose as coffee but black tea does have some caffeine. Caffeine by itself will stimulate the nervous system but will also put a body in a state of anxiety or fight or flight response. It comes with elevated cortisol and adrenaline, hypoglycemia, jitters, the increased heart rate and feelings of anxiety.

L-theanine affects the brain also but in a different way and actually in a number of different ways. Acting as an anxiolytic, it is known to amplify alpha brain waves, allowing for a type of calm alertness and even heightened creativity. Theanine has also been shown to boost levels of GABA, as well as other hormones and compounds that promote calm, focus, regulated mood, and more. By itself, l-theanine is an effective nootropic. But when combined with caffeine there's a pronounced synergistic effect. This means you experience heightened focus, awareness, and energy, as well as reduced stress and improved mental endurance, to even higher levels. What does l-theanine exactly do to our brain? The easy way to determine is to give some tea to subjects in an experiment and then hook up their brain to the electroencephalograph, the EEG machine, to measure their brain waves patterns (L-theanine, a natural constituent in tea, and its effect on mental state. Asia Pac J Clin Nutr. 2008;17 Suppl 1:167-8). There are four mental states or frequency waves that our brain is producing. Delta at around 0.3 to 3 Hz that is a deep sleep state. Then theta 4-7 Hz that is light sleep. It is a state when we are dreaming. Then alpha 8-13 HZ that is normal relaxed awaken state. It is a state of for example relaxed meditation. And then there is a beta at 14 hertz that is anxiety awaken state. We spend most of our waking life in a beta state. If you have a job to do or have to cross the street and don't want to get hit by a car you want to be in a beta state. If you are relaxed on a beach then alpha is more pleasing. But because of caffeine or other stimulants or general stress and anxiety, most people lose the ability to go into the relaxed alpha state. After tea consumption, we can see a brain shifting to an alpha activity in a potent manner. 50 mg of l-theanine or 2 cups of green tea is all it takes for a significant effect on the general state of mental alertness. L-theanine could also help people relax before bedtime, get to sleep more easily, and sleep more deeply. It would not be a good idea to drink a black tea before bedtime because of the caffeine but rather a green tea. In the morning a black tea would be more beneficial because of the synergistic effect of a low dose of caffeine with a calming effect of l-theanine. L-theanine may improve a person's attention and reaction times and in combination with caffeine, it may lead to improvements in alertness as well. Keep in mind that if you take supplements there is green tea extract that is more potent as an antioxidant and separately there is l-theanine. If you drink tea then you will get both. The most powerful green tea is actually not a tea at all but whole leaves powder that is dissolved in water and then consumed called matcha tea. When we throw away tea leaves after making the tea we are essentially throwing away nutrition. When we drink matcha tea we don't drink tea at all but eat whole tea leaves in a powdered form. It was invented in China about a thousand years ago and then it spread to Japan. Also, there is one more thing to have in mind. Tea from China depending on a local area where it is grown can be polluted by lead because there is a lot of air pollution there so some tea might have elevated heavy metals level. Tea from Japan and other places so far is tested to be pure.

If we look at the list, we will see that just below green tea extract is the coffee cherry (Cascara) powder with an ORAC value of 343,900. It is a very potent antioxidant source and it is commercially available. It is used to make a tea. What is a potency of this tea as an antioxidant I don't know. I wasn't able to find much research on it. The caffeine content of Cáscara has been reported to be significantly lower than coffee or tea, with 50mg of caffeine present in a 300ml serving of cascara tea. Next in the line is sumac bran with 312,400. This is not sumac but a sumac bran. The bran is the portion of the grain that is processed out of the grain to make ingredients like white flour for example. As far as I have seen this is not commercially available. Same with the sorghum bran. There is a sumac bran organic extract supplement that is commercially available. It supposedly has an ORAC value above 15 million units per 100 grams. If you don't want bran extract you can still find regular whole food sumac spice. It is a popular spice in Middle Eastern cuisine. It has a red color and taste that could best be described as a salty lemon. In fact, the saltiness taste is so strong it makes an excellent sodium-free alternative. If you've ever dined in a Middle Eastern restaurant, you may have noticed the dark red powder that dusts everything from salads to meat to baklava. That is it. When you look and go down at the list you will notice that most of the items will be different spices or herbs. Rosemary, meadowsweet, peppermint, thyme, wild marjoram, cinnamon, turmeric, lemon balm, sage, allspice, oregano and so on. Most of these spices and herbs will be used in normal cooking but only in small amounts and sporadically. Sometimes even a pinch of them will have an impact on overall levels of consumed antioxidants. If we want a real increase in our antioxidant intake realistically it would be a hard time doing it with just spices and herbs. What we can do is to use them as a supplement. For example, you can mix turmeric and ground pepper and amla and take a teaspoon of it every day with water as a supplement. That will be a more significant increase in antioxidant intake instead of eating curry as a spice with a meal. There is a long list of potent spices and some are stronger than others but there is a question of their antioxidant bioavailability.

If we want to see real in vivo results on the effect of spices to see what they do and if they do anything in doses that are used in normal cooking, we can look at some studies. In this study (Bioavailability of herbs and spices in humans as determined by ex vivo inflammatory suppression and DNA strand breaks. J Am Coll Nutr. 2012 Aug;31(4):288-94) they feed subjects with different types of spices for a week. The quantity they used and this is very important is just a small amount that people get in a normal diet like for example 0.3 grams of cloves or up to 2.8 grams of ginger. They used just 0.3 grams of turmeric per day, 0.3 g/day of cayenne pepper, 1.7 g/day of paprika, 1.7 g/day of Saigon cinnamon, 2.8 g/day of cumin, Mediterranean oregano 1.1 g/day, black pepper 2.8 g/day, rosemary 2.8 g/day, dalmatian sage 1.7 g/day, clove 0.3 g/day and ginger 2.8 g/day. After a week, they drew blood and then dropped that blood onto human white blood cells that had been exposed to oxidized cholesterol. Then researchers measured how much inflammatory cytokines white blood cells produced in response. They wanted to see how much eating different spices will lower inflammatory response and also how much will they protect DNA. This is the closest as we can get to measure the real-life influence of some food because they did not just measure the antioxidant level in the blood or they did not just use a spice like for example turmeric and measure its effects directly. They used the blood of people that have been eating spices in realistic dosages. The result was that cloves, ginger, rosemary, and turmeric were able to significantly stifle the inflammatory response while black pepper, cayenne, cinnamon, cumin, oregano, paprika, sage, and heated turmeric did nothing. They also measured the impact on DNA damage. Paprika, rosemary, ginger, heat-treated turmeric, sage, and cumin protected against DNA strand breaks. This does not automatically mean that other spices are useless and not bioavailable. There is a possibility of that. It means two things, they might not be bioavailable or that dosages were low to elicit an effect. In regards to DNA protection in normal conditions, people will have 7 to 10 percent of their DNA in tissue samples damaged. Body repairs damage all the time and some DNA damage in 7 to 10 cells on every 100 cells is considered normal. Usually, people that have a bad diet have around 10 percent. In the study, ginger has broth down this number from 10 to 8, rosemary to 7 and turmeric to 4.5. Just a small pinch of 0.3 grams of turmeric was able to bring down DNA damage in half. This is for a heat-treated turmeric, the raw turmeric showed no effect while exactly the opposite was found for anti-inflammatory effect. Heat-treated turmeric showed no effect on inflammation while raw powder did. It seems that we should consume both forms of turmeric. This result means that antioxidants and in this case spices and especially turmeric have an ability to prolong life.

Back in a day when I first started incorporating this knowledge into my life, I started with a basic mix of turmeric powder and ground black pepper. I didn't take any of the supplements I just used ground turmeric powder that I purchased in a regular health food store. At a beginning that was all I did. Every morning I took one teaspoon of turmeric and black pepper mix. Later when I learned more about nutrition, I started to change some of my grocery decisions. I have already been eating mostly vegan whole food healthy diet but I still managed to increase substantially the level of antioxidant that I consume. For people that don't want to do this and that still want to eat oil and meat and sugar and all of the rest of the unhealthy foods, one easy step will be to do what I did. Just go to the health food store and get some turmeric. The next step for me was to add other potent sources into the recipe. The amount of turmeric we can safely consume in not that large. The upper limit is about 10 grams per day because it has high amounts of bioavailable oxalic acid and also it will start to actually damage our DNA if we overconsume it. The safe upper limit for most of the people is 10 grams but 5 grams of it is an optimal dose. To increase the potency of the recipe without increasing turmeric to unhealthy levels I added other antioxidants to the mix that were found to decrease inflammation in the study I referenced. I added dried ginger, rosemary, and cloves that I got from a health food store as well. This was my recipe for a couple of years until a discovered the research behind amla and then added amla as well. This doesn't mean you should do this if you are happy with just turmeric than go with that or you can make your own recipe. This is the mixture that I created on the basis of clinical studies for myself. Today I take 10 to 15 grams of this mix every morning and this will give me a value of around 10,000 to 20,000 ORAC units. One spoon of this mixture will have more antioxidants than what average American that eats a standard American diet will consume in a whole week. Plus, on top of antioxidants, there are other phytochemicals in there as well that have beneficial properties from the immune system, cognitive function, endocrine function and so on and because this is a whole food mixture there will be a food synergy effect as well. The best thing about this is that you can make this "supplement" yourself and it is dirt cheap. If you don't want to do anything in regard to your health and diet and don't want to change anything then just do this one thing. It will benefit you more than any other health intervention. The worst thing about this is taste. It is very nasty. The way I do it I just put it directly into my mouth and then I drink water and swallow. I tried to mix it in with the juice or water or in tea, and it didn't help. As soon as it hits any type of liquid it starts to soak up and then it will bulk up and will release all of its taste to that liquid making it even worse. After I created this form of the antioxidant rich herbal mix, I created one more.

There are essential oils that are very potent antioxidants like clove essential oil. I decided to mix them and make an antioxidant rich essential oil mix for consumption. These oils are so potent that they will create burns and cannot be consumed without diluting and I didn't want to just mix them with olive oil. I used black cumin seed oil as a base. It is potent oil by itself and even swallowing black seed oil can sometimes lead to digestive problems, such as stomach upset, constipation, and vomiting. That is the reason why you should never overconsume it. One teaspoon is all we need. In traditional medicine, black cumin seed oil has been used for thousands of years from India to the Middle East to ancient Greece. Black cumin ranks among the most popular herbs in the history of medicine. In ancient civilizations, it was used to improve digestion and in the treatment of colds, headaches, infections, and toothache. Black cumin seeds were even found in pharaoh Tutankhamun's tomb for use in the afterlife. Due to its strengthening properties physicians like Hippocrates prescribed it to patients who experienced general illness and feebleness. Even the Prophet Muhammad of Islam supposedly stated that the black cumin seed is a cure for every known disease except death. This seed is also known as the "seed of blessing" in the Holy Bible. In 1996, due to its proven chemopreventive and chemotherapeutic properties, the US Food and Drug Administration approved the use of black cumin in the treatment of cancerous diseases. Out of the vast number of active phytochemicals in the oil, the most effective are nigellone that relaxes muscles and expands bronchial tubes and thymoquinone that enhances the secretion of bile, lowers excessive acidity, reduces cholesterol, and helps with digestive problems. The beneficial effect of black cumin has also been proven in the treatment of dermatological problems: eczema, skin fungus, and acne. Due to its strong antibacterial effect, black cumin oil helps in the treatment of influenza. In a nutshell, there is an exceptionally broad spectrum of its beneficial health effects but we are going to use it because it is a powerful antioxidant that can be taken directly without danger of irritation. And we are using it here as a base in which we are going to add other more potent oils. Not all essential oils are edible. If you want to add them you will have to do the research yourself for every type of essential oil that you want. Some essential oils, in the same manner as herbal teas, should not be mixed together because they might have adverse reactions. This is a complicated subject and I will not go into depth here. Some general rule of thumb is that if the plant is edible like for example cloves, then essential oil from that plant will be edible as well. Clove oil is a superstar with a nice smell and taste and an ORAC score of more than a million. There is also one more issue. Some edible oils are also toxic because they are much more concentrated chemically then a plant that they are created of and if there is some toxin in that plant it will be much more prominent in the oil. Nutmeg is a good example. Nutmeg tastes great in cookies and eggnog, but too much can cause hallucinations. It has amphetamine-like substance in it (Christmas gingerbread (Lebkuchen) and Christmas cheer--review of the potential role of mood elevating amphetamine-like compounds formed in vivo and in furno. Prague Med Rep. 2005;106(1):27-38). The toxic dose of nutmeg for an adult is two teaspoons and for the essential oil is basically zero. Children who get into the container and people who deliberately swallow a lot of nutmeg trying to get high will be able to achieve hallucinations but also will become miserably sick. Nausea, vomiting, agitation, prolonged drowsiness, and coma are all possible. In the Middle Ages nutmeg was used as an abortifacient so eating nutmeg essential oil is quite dangerous especially by a pregnant woman and children. It is truthful that in most of the cases oil is the less toxic option then the nut because most of the toxins present in the nuts don't get extracted when the oil is steam distilled from the nuts, but the elemicin and myristicin, the two psychoactive substances in the nutmeg are extracted. Even a tiny drop of 0.25 ml of 100% pure therapeutic grade nutmeg oil will give you a mild trip with visuals, euphoria, etc. Even handling nutmeg oil can be dangerous because you can lick your fingers unintentionally. The effects begin in about 30 minutes and peak after about 3-5 hours. Oil of wintergreen is another example and it is just a name for methyl salicylate, a relative of aspirin (acetylsalicylic acid). Small amounts are safe to use as flavoring agents, but the bottle must be locked up, where children can't get to it. Small amounts of oil of wintergreen can poison children. Because the oil of wintergreen is rapidly absorbed, children can become dangerously ill very quickly. Peppermint is used for gastrointestinal discomfort. It's important to choose the correct species of mint, as some types are poisonous; for example, pennyroyal oil is very poisonous to the liver. Eucalyptus is used for its soothing effects when inhaled, for example during a cold or cough. If swallowed, eucalyptus oil can cause seizures. Sage oil has been used as a scent, seasoning, and remedy. Swallowing more than a very small amount has caused seizures in children. Camphor is used as a moth repellent and as an ingredient in skin preparations. Even a small amount of camphor is dangerous if swallowed. Seizures can begin within a few minutes. Camphor poisoning also occurred when skin preparations containing camphor were applied repeatedly on children. If you want to make antioxidant health promoting oil mix supplement start with black cumin seed oil and add clove oil and oil of wild oregano and then go from there. Do the research for every essential oil you want to add. There is a lot of phytochemicals in essential oils besides antioxidants that will have biological reactions in the body or even drug interactions. You need to know exactly what they are and what effect they can possibly have or you risk health implications. You shouldn't use essential oils in early pregnancy at all until more research is conducted on the topic.

The list of ORAC values of essential oils is as follow:

1.	Clove	1,078,700	37.	Tarragon	37,900
2.	Myrrh	379,800	38.	Peppermint	37,300
3.	Citronella	312,000	39.	Cardamom	36,500
4.	Coriander	298,300	40.	Dill	35,600
5.	Fennel	238,400	41.	Celery Seed	30,300
6.	Clary Sage	221,000	42.	Mandarin	26,500
7.	German Chamomile	218,600	43.	Lime	26,200
8.	Cedarwood	169,000	44.	Galbanum	26,200
9.	Rose	158,100	45.	Myrtle	25,400
10.	Nutmeg	158,100	46.	Cypress	24,300
11.	Marjoram	151,000	47.	Grapefruit	22,600
12.	Melissa	139,905	48.	Hyssop	20,900
13.	Ylang	134,300	49.	Balsam Fir	20,500
14.	Palmarosa	130,000	50.	Niaouli	18,600
15.	Rosewood	113,200	51.	Thyme	15,960
16.	Manuka	106,200	52.	Oregano	15,300
17.	Wintergreen	101,800	53.	Cassia	15,170
18.	Geranium	101,000	54.	Sage	14,800
19.	Ginger	99,300	55.	Mountain Savory	11,300
20.	Bay Laurel	98,900	56.	Cinnamon Bark	10,340
21.	Eucalyptus Citriodora	83,000	57.	Tsuga	7,100
22.	Cumin	82,400	58.	Valerian	6,200
23.	Black Pepper	79,700	59.	Cistus	3,860
24.	Vetiver	74,300	60.	Eucalyptus Globulus	2,410
25.	Petitgrain	73,600	61.	Orange	1,890
26.	Blue Cypress	73,100	62.	Lemongrass	1,780

27.	Citrus Hystrix	69,200	63.	Helichrysum	1,740
28.	Douglas Fir	69,000	64.	Ravensara	890
29.	Blue Tansy	68,800	65.	Lemon	660
30.	Goldenrod	61,900	66.	Frankincense	630
31.	Melaleuca ericifolia	61,100	67.	Spearmint	540
32.	Blue Yarrow	55,900	68.	Lavender	360
33.	Spikenard	54,800	69.	Rosemary	330
34.	Basil	54,000	70.	Juniper	250
35.	Patchouli	49,400	71.	Roman Chamomile	240
36.	White Fir	47,900	72.	Sandalwood	160

Keep in mind that this is a value for 100mg and it would be hard to consume 100mg of these types of oils because they are very potent and could create a range of health issues if overconsumed from vomiting and nausea to seizures and coma. Light and oxygen degrade these oils. Presumably, these tests used fresh sources that had been exposed to minimal air and light. Essential oils break down relatively fast upon exposure to the atmosphere, heat, and light. It's why they are stored in amber or dark-colored glass bottles. Air exposure causes the metabolites to become oxidized and rancid. If you have oils that you opened many months ago that have not constantly been kept tightly sealed in a cool and dark place such as a drawer, it's likely the ORAC is much lower. In that scenario, they may actually be rancid. If that's the case, it's time to replace it. One more consideration is that some oils don't mix because they have adverse effects. Me personally just use clove and oil of wild oregano mixed in into black cumin seed oil and I take one teaspoon of it a day on top of the herbal mix. I take one teaspoon of oil and one regular spoon of my herbal mix and together they have more than 30,000 units on an ORAC scale. If I don't do anything else this will be enough to provide me with an adequate level of antioxidant intake but I do eat healthy and do drink herbal tea and green tea and take some antioxidant supplements on top of that like astaxanthin. In the mentioned study I was actually a little surprised that for example cinnamon and oregano showed no benefit in the fighting inflammation. There were a number of health studies on both of them that did show a significant health effect. I can only speculate that the dose was low.

In this study (The radioprotective effects of Origanum vulgare extract against genotoxicity induced by (131)I in human blood lymphocyte. doi:

10.1089/cbr.2012.1284) researchers measured the protective effect of oregano on DNA damaging effect of radiation. Radioactive iodine is used in people that have overactive thyroid glands or thyroid cancer. Thyroid glands will absorb that radioactive iodine and that will destroy part of the gland, but also as a consequence radiation exposure will increase the risk of developing new cancers in the rest of the body later on. Treatment is effective but it is dangerous as well. Researchers tested the ability of oregano to protect chromosomes of human blood cells in vitro from exposure to radioactive iodine. The addition of oregano extract managed to reduce radioactive damage as much as 70 percent. There are other studies that also found beneficial effects of oregano. In this study (Anticancer Activity of Certain Herbs and Spices on the Cervical Epithelial Carcinoma (HeLa) Cell Line. doi: 10.1155/2012/564927) oregano was able to beat out all but bay leaves in its ability to suppress cervical cancer cell growth in vitro while leaving normal cells alone. They compered extracts of oregano, bay leaves, fennel, lavender, paprika, parsley, rosemary, and thyme. Oil of oregano beside its antioxidant properties and anti-cancer properties is one of the nature most powerful antibiotics. It contains carvacrol and thymol, two antibacterial and antifungal compounds. In fact, research shows oregano oil is effective against many clinical strains of bacteria, including Escherichia coli and Pseudomonas aeruginosa both of which are common causes of the urinary tract and respiratory tract infections. In studies it was shown to be as effective as antibiotics (Effects of Essential Oils and Monolaurin on Staphylococcus aureus: In Vitro and In Vivo Studies. doi: 10.1080/15376520590968833). Besides bacteria, it also kills fungi and viruses. A test-tube study of the effectiveness of oregano oil on 16 different strains of Candida concluded that oregano oil may be a good alternative treatment for Candida yeast infections (In vitro activity of origanum vulgare essential oil against candida species. doi: 10.1590/S1517-83820100001000018). Research has also shown that oregano oil may be effective against types of bacteria that can become resistant to antibiotics. It is very potent. The only question still unanswered is does the oregano oil kills all types of bacteria or is selective? Antibiotics will kill everything and will make havoc in our gastrointestinal tract killing both good and bad bacteria but the oil of oregano might not be as bad. There are some indications that it would not be as toxic to probiotic bacteria as regular antibiotics and if this is correct it would make oil of oregano a superior product to regular antibiotics. I want to mention here also that you do not take oil of oregano as a substitute to already prescribed therapy and always consult your doctor before you do anything. If you are sick you need to take medicine, consider oil of oregano as a form of preventive medicine or as an addition to your already prescribed medications. Never do anything on your own.

One additional good source of antioxidants is cinnamon. It didn't show an anti-inflammatory effect in the study but it does have an ORAC value of 131,420. The amount used in a study was 1.7 grams. From all spices in the world, it is second in popularity behind black pepper. It is a bark of different types of Cinnamomum trees. There's Ceylon, Chinese cinnamon, Vietnamese cinnamon, and Indonesian cinnamon. They are all potent antioxidants. The good thing about cinnamon is not just its antioxidant power, it has other benefits as well. It is very good for blood sugar control. " The available in vitro and animal in vivo evidence suggests that cinnamon has anti-inflammatory, antimicrobial, antioxidant, antitumor, cardiovascular, cholesterol-lowering, and immunomodulatory effects. In vitro studies have demonstrated that cinnamon may act as an insulin-mimetic, to potentiate insulin activity or to stimulate cellular glucose metabolism. Furthermore, animal studies have demonstrated strong hypoglycemic properties." (Cinnamon and health. doi: 10.1080/10408390902773052). But there is a catch. From all types of cinnamon with beneficial antioxidant properties Chinese cinnamon, also known as cassia cinnamon was found to have a toxic effect on a liver. It is because of a substance called coumarin that was banned as a food additive. It was not found in Ceylon and there is no data for the other two but in most of the markets, there are only Ceylon or Cassia that are sold. In the US you can find both types and both are labeled cinnamon. If it is not specially labeled as Ceylon it is Chinese because it is cheaper. There is no upper tolerable limit for Ceylon and if you want you can add as much as you desire but if you use Chinese Cassia then you should not exceed 5 grams in a day. Children consuming just a quarter of a teaspoon two times a week are at risk of toxicity. The solution is to switch to Ceylon and that will negate the toxicity except there is a catch. The same substance coumarin that is toxic to the liver is what gives cinnamon its diabetes fighting properties. All studies that have ever shown blood sugar benefits were done on Cassia and all other studies that were done on other types of cinnamon never showed any type of benefit (Ceylon cinnamon does not affect postprandial plasma glucose or insulin in subjects with impaired glucose tolerance. doi: 10.1017/S0007114511005113). If you want antioxidant benefits without blood sugar control benefits you can switch to Ceylon. If you want you might try to combine both types of cinnamon. Use a safe amount of Cassia with the addition of Ceylon. But how effective is cinnamon for a blood sugar control anyway? The effect is modest to a strong, something in a line of metformin. Metformin (Glucophage) is the first line of medication for type 2 diabetes and cinnamon can rival its effectiveness. In a practical sense if you consume cinnamon before glucose tolerance test you can significantly lower the glucose spike and essentially cheat the test. You would need 5 grams or at least a teaspoon of cinnamon to have an effect. One half of a teaspoon is not enough. A half teaspoon a day is where you want to be if you have a healthy liver and want to use cinnamon for a blood sugar control prevention (Cinnamon intake lowers fasting blood glucose: meta-analysis. doi: 10.1089/jmf.2010.0180). It will give you a positive effect on blood sugar and other health benefits without stressing the liver too much. If you just want a taste and antioxidant properties then go with Ceylon.

Besides cinnamon, one more herb that has high antioxidant value can be problematic and you should be aware of this not to overdo with it. Peppermint has an ability to interfere with hormones in the body and it can have testosterone lowering effect (Effects of peppermint teas on plasma testosterone, follicle-stimulating hormone, and luteinizing hormone levels and testicular tissue in rats. Urology. 2004 Aug;64(2):394-8). If you are men this would not be so beneficial but if you are a woman with polycystic ovarian syndrome spearmint has potential as a treatment (Role of Essential Oil of Mentha Spicata (Spearmint) in Addressing Reverse Hormonal and Folliculogenesis Disturbances in a Polycystic Ovarian Syndrome in a Rat Model doi: 10.15171/apb.2017.078). Peppermint can help with PCOS through inhibition of testosterone and restoration of follicular development in ovarian tissue. It has antiandrogen properties and significantly decreases testosterone level and hirsutism in women with PCOS but be careful, it will do the same in women without PCOS and men as well. Don't overdo it, it is a strong antioxidant but there are other antioxidants that don't have adverse effects. Peppermint has one unique ability to fight off nausea but ginger can do that as well. If we look at all herbal teas, in my opinion, there are much more superior choices and the number one from all beverages and the herbal tea with the highest antioxidant value is hibiscus tea.

I wasn't able to find an ORAC value for dried hibiscus flower all I was able to find is ORAC for already brewed tea and it is the highest value from all beverages. ORAC value for brewed hibiscus tea is 6,990. Keep in mind that this is for 100g of tea and usually serving size for tea is one cup. One cup has 236 grams and usually uses one teabag for one cup in normal tea preparation. One cup per bag is a good rule of thumb and as a standard that is used in laboratory research. Because the tea bag contains 2-3 grams of tea you will usually get very weak tea that has a light color. Nevertheless that 3 grams of grounded hibiscus browed in a 236ml of water gives an ORAC score of 6,990 per 100 grams. The whole cup of hibiscus tea will have around 15,400 units. It is one of the sources of antioxidants that have very strong red pigment with very high potency and the source that is cheap and easily available. It also tastes good unlike some of the spices. You can mix hibiscus in different dishes as well, you don't have to use it just like a tea. What I do I buy it on bulk in a health food store. I will grind it in a coffee grinder and then use it as a powder for cereal or some other dish. If you add it to the cereal, for example, it gives a blueberry flavor and a red color. But if you just want a tea that is a good option as well. What I do is that I don't use teabags. I use hibiscus from a health food store that comes in a bulk and then I put as much as I feel is needed. Usually, I will make 2 cups of tea with different herbal teas but also I will add one whole tablespoon of hibiscus powder per cup. That is about 15 to 20 grams of it. If tea bag has 3 grams and I am adding 20 that is 6 times as much. In theory, this should give a whopping 35,000 units on the ORAC scale even without counting other herbs that I will add as well. My hibiscus tea is dark red in color and in some cases almost black and it is more powerful then slightly colored standardly prepared hibiscus tea. These numbers are all speculation because I wasn't able to find ORAC value for dried hibiscus powder so I am using the data that I have and the numbers may be wrong but at the end of the day hibiscus is one of the easiest and one of the most potent natural pigments that are available and will boost antioxidant value of diet significantly. It is the most antioxidant rich tea, even more so then matcha tea. And it is one of the antioxidants that is not just powerful but also completely bioavailable (Consumption of Hibiscus sabdariffa L. aqueous extract and its impact on systemic antioxidant potential in healthy subjects. doi: 10.1002/jsfa.5615). One cup was able to create a significant rise in the antioxidant blood potential of human subjects. One of the effects of hibiscus tea consumption is the lowering of blood pressure. It is a side effect free natural medicine for hypertension. A cup of hibiscus tea with each meal was able to lower blood pressure by 7 points at average (Hibiscus sabdariffa L. tea (tisane) lowers blood pressure in prehypertensive and mildly hypertensive adults. doi: 10.3945/jn.109.115097). This study lasted for 6 weeks without any other form of intervention in subjects that did not take any other blood pressure lowering medications previously. Two cups a day every morning was able to rival a leading blood-pressure drug, captopril (Effectiveness and tolerability of a standardized extract from Hibiscus sabdariffa in patients with mild to moderate hypertension: a controlled and randomized clinical trial. Phytomedicine. 2004 Jul;11(5):375-82). They were using a total of 5 tea bags for those two cups and that was enough to rival a starting dose of 25mg of captopril taken twice a day. We still need to remember that there is no cure for cardiovascular disease other than vegan, no cholesterol, a low saturated fat diet with exercise, so don't think that taking high antioxidant rich foods will save you from stroke or heart attack. It is better than nothing and if you don't want to change your diet and lifestyle then do at least incorporate hibiscus tea and other antioxidant rich foods. Even the food industry tried to add hibiscus extract to meat and was conducting a line of hibiscus extract experiments. They wanted to create "health promoting" meat that they would be able to market as a new discovery of science. They tried with acai extract first but that failed because of the color (Protein oxidation in emulsified cooked burger patties with added fruit extracts: Influence on color and texture deterioration during chill storage. doi: 10.1016/j.meatsci.2010.02.008). Hibiscus has pure red pigment so it would be more useful but that failed also because of the taste. The taste was not compatible and eventually, the industry gave up the idea at least publicly. What usually happens in industry funded research is that if the experiment fails, they just completely ignore the findings and in most cases don't even publish the research at all. The cigarette industry, for example, tried to add acai to cigarettes for lung cancer and emphysema prevention in smoking mice. Emphysema kills and has no cure and people with this condition have to quit smoking or risk death and that is bad for business so they tried to add antioxidants to cigarettes directly. I am not kidding here is the study (Addition of açaí (Euterpe oleracea) to cigarettes has a protective effect against emphysema in mice. doi: 10.1016/j.fct.2010.12.007). The conclusion of the study was: " The presence of açai extract in cigarettes had a protective effect against emphysema in mice, probably by reducing oxidative and inflammatory reactions. These results raise the possibility that addition of açaí extract to normal cigarettes could reduce their harmful effects." So far there is only one side effect from hibiscus tea that I am aware of and that is the erosion of tooth enamel. Hibiscus tea has strong acids in it and it has the ability to erode enamel. It is the same with other acidic fruits and vegetables as well, for example, citrus, so this is nothing unique to hibiscus. Coca Cola can do this also and it is actually one of the most acidic drinks out there with a pH of around 2.5. There is a simple fix you can do and that is to swish mouth with water to clear the acid after drinking it. Or use a straw. Is there an upper limit of how much you can drink or any form of toxicity associated with it? The answer is yes and no. The only possible issue with hibiscus tea is its high manganese content. One cup of hibiscus tea has 1.130 mg of manganese which is 49% of RDA. And this is for normal low potency regular tea. If you drink stronger tea it is probable that you will get 100% or more of RDA of manganese in just one cup so the only question is the level of toxicity of manganese and how much can you consume without creating a problem? Usually, people don't get manganese deficiency because it is a mineral that is abundant in plants. Also, the manganese is absorbed better when intake is low. The tolerable upper intake level is 11 mg per day for adults 19 and older and this is well above 2,2 mg of RDA. This is the official recommendation that is conservative. A healthy person with functioning liver and kidneys should be able to excrete excess dietary manganese without creating a terrible issue but if you go above 11 mg in a prolonged period of time it can have a negative effect especially to the brain. Exposure to toxic levels of manganese will cause clinical signs and symptoms resembling Parkinson's disease. Manganese toxicity has been associated with dopaminergic dysfunction but so far this condition is found only in people that were exposed to it by environmental factors like inhaling inorganic manganese for example. It is highly unlikely that you will be able to megadose yourself in such a toxic level with food. So far in all studies with dietary manganese, the levels in the blood were stable even with dietary manganese that exceeded RDA. In this study (Dietary manganese intake and type of lipid do not affect clinical or neuropsychological measures in healthy young women. J Nutr. 2003 Sep;133(9):2849-56) dietary intake of manganese was

20 mg for 8 weeks and it didn't result in toxicity signs. So how much hibiscus is safe? I will say as much as you want if you have healthy liver and kidneys and you are not a child. To be on a safe side if you drink up to five cups a day there should be any toxicity.

One more excellent source of antioxidants is cocoa powder. It has an ORAC value of 55,653 which if compared to other more potent sources might not seem as much. Keep in mind that you can only consume small amounts of spices and herbs but you can easily eat an entire 70% cocoa black chocolate that will give an ORAC value of about 38,500. Don't think now that milk chocolate is healthy and a good source of antioxidants as well. It is not because of the milk. Milk protein binds to and will stop the absorption of polyphenols from the cacao bean and milk chocolate has much less actual cocoa in the first place and much more sugar and saturated fat. Milk will stop the absorption of phytochemicals in tea as well and dairy products in general do this because of the milk protein. It is casein (milk protein) that is a problem so avoiding any form of dairy with high antioxidant rich food is the necessity if you want to have the normal levels of antioxidant absorption. For example, if you make hot cocoa with milk or cream instead of nut milk or water or even if you eat dark chocolate and then drink a cup of milk the antioxidant effects will be suppressed. "Addition of milk either during injestion, or in the manufacturing process, therefore inhibits the in vivo antioxidant activity of chocolate and the absorption into the bloodstream of the epicatechin" (Plasma antioxidants from chocolate. Nature. 2003 Aug 28;424(6952):1013). Dark chocolate is the only choice if you want to reap the antioxidant benefits from cocoa. Unprocessed cocoa powder is even better. There is no real raw cocoa in reality. All cocoa is processed and when you process food it loses some of the nutrients. Raw cocoa powder is just less processed and will have more antioxidants somewhere in the range of 80,000. Normally processed cocoa powder will be around 50,000 and milk chocolate and candy are basically useless and should be avoided because of all of the sugar and fat. The reason why cocoa is considered a superfood is because of its nutrient density. When cacao beans are processed to create cocoa powder one of the steps involves removing the fat out of the bean. It is one of the rare cases in the food industry where the fat is actually removed to create the finished product. When you remove the fat from the bean you are left with antioxidants, minerals, fiber, vitamins, protein and all other nutrients in the cocoa powder and cocoa butter on the other side. Cocoa butter is an empty calorie and is added back later when chocolate is made so this will negate any of the increases in nutrient profile but if you consume cocoa powder then you essentially have a super nutrient dense food source that is one of the most if not the most nutrient dense food on the planet. Dark chocolate is better than milk chocolate and other sweets but even dark chocolate has added fat and sugar. Cocoa butter is one of the rare sources of saturated fat in the plant kingdom and is best to be avoided. Other sources will be palm tree oil and coconut oil. Saturated fat and lard are the same molecules. Saturated fat from plant or animal kingdom is bad for us. Lard is worse because lard will also create inflammation while coconut oil or cocoa butter will not but will still have negative effects on insulin sensitivity, the brain, the arteries and will still raise bad cholesterol. Saturated fat is better to be avoided in excessive amounts even if it comes from the plant kingdom. If you eat animal products you are already eating too much fat. Even if the meat is lean there is still fat inside the muscle tissue that you don't see. Go with the cocoa powder. If you want higher potency then go with "raw" cocoa powder, it will have 30% more antioxidants then regular processed powder. And on top of that cocoa taste good. Cocoa powder is especially rich in minerals and especially magnesium that most people don't get enough, to begin with. 100 grams of cocoa powder will have 499 mg of magnesium. It will give 3.837 mg of manganese which is 183% of RDA, 105% of phosphorus, 72% for zinc and so on. Because there is not enough magnesium in animal products and most population don't eat enough greens adding cocoa powder to a diet will have beneficial effects even if we disregard its antioxidant profile. Preventing magnesium deficiency with one dark chocolate a day or even better, adding cocoa powder to a smoothie or just drinking hot cocoa will have significant health effects in the long run if you are deficient with magnesium. When we look at the antioxidant content of raw cocoa beans, they contain approximately 6–8% polyphenols by dry weight. That is one of the best sources of antioxidants in nature. When the fat is removed to create cocoa powder polyphenols content will go well above 10% by dry weight. If we look at the clinical research and what is scientifically shown to be a benefit from coco consumption we will find a lot of research. The problem is that most of that research is funded by the chocolate producing companies to boost the health claims of their products as a marketing strategy not necessarily as scientific exploration. But still, there is a lot of independent research as well. It has proven beneficial cardiovascular properties (The emerging role of flavonoid-rich cocoa and chocolate in cardiovascular health and disease. Nutr Rev. 2006 Mar;64(3):109-18). It is as with any other antioxidant rich food, these antioxidant flavonoids in cocoa will help to lower blood pressure and inflammation. Cocoa will also lower bad cholesterol but also will help to boost the good cholesterol and will suppress the oxidation of LDL (Plasma LDL and HDL cholesterol and oxidized LDL concentrations are altered in normal and hypercholesterolemic humans after intake of different levels of cocoa powder. J Nutr. 2007 Jun;137(6):1436-41). Cholesterol lowering medication usually only blocks the production of bad cholesterol in the liver and cannot do anything to help to increase the production of good cholesterol. At the same time, cocoa also helps to reduce platelet reactivity and it helps to open up coronary arteries (Dark chocolate improves coronary vasomotion and reduces platelet reactivity. Circulation. 2007 Nov

20;116(21):2376-82). It will help with cholesterol, boost the immune system, unstiffen the arteries, lower the inflammation, provide a good amount of magnesium and other minerals and fiber. Besides all of this and regular antioxidant benefits that it will provide there is one unique health promoting effect of cocoa. Epicatechin has an ability to lower the myostatin levels. Epicatechin is a naturally occurring phytochemical present in dark chocolate and cacao. If you are familiar with bodybuilding you will know very well what myostatin is. Myostatin inhibitors are not on the market yet but it is believed to be the next big thing in the pharmaceutical industry, something so big that it will rival the discovery of antibiotics. Currently, there are billions of dollars spent every year into research on myostatin inhibition. Myostatin's primary function in the body is to inhibit muscle growth. Myostatin acts in direct opposition to another protein, follistatin, which functions to increase muscle growth. Inhibiting myostatin will benefit elderly people, people with aids and other muscle wasting diseases and the best thing of all it will benefit the food industry. Today farmers use finaplex implants for cattle that are filled with trenbolone acetate and also use other steroids to promote muscle grow and increase nutritional partitioning so that they can have bigger cattle. Myostatin inhibition, if ever discovered, will bring revolution into farming. In humans, it will make bodybuilding and other muscle wasting diseases obsolete. Before there are drugs on the market with potential side-effects the epicatechin from cocoa is proven to be able to both inhibit myostatin and boost follistatin (Effects of epicatechin on molecular modulators of skeletal muscle growth and differentiation. doi: 10.1016/j.jnutbio.2013.09.007). "The flavanol epicatechin (Epi) enhances exercise capacity in mice and Epi-rich cocoa improves skeletal muscle structure in heart failure patients. Epicatechin may thus, hold promise as treatment for sarcopenia." Myostatin levels increase during aging and this is actually the primal reason why sarcopenia is happening. It is not lowering of androgenic hormones that is the main cause, it is one of the reasons but an increase in myostatin levels is the main one. My advice is to exercise daily and drink cocoa daily. There is only one thing that we need to keep in mind and that is that cocoa has 230mg of caffeine in 100 grams of powder. It is not a good idea to drink it or eat chocolate before bedtime.

Besides spices, essential oils, herbs, and supplements what are some other good sources of antioxidants in general? Some fruits are better than others, some vegetables are better than others. If we look at the fruits the different types of berries, in general, are the richest source. Plums, apples, cherries are also good. Fruit depending on fructose content can have a high antioxidant value per calorie and also we can eat a lot of fruit at a single sitting, unlike spices or herbs. One pound of raw plums for example that are not from Amazon rain forest like acai and are not as expensive will have 210 calories and around 30,000 units on an ORAC scale. Average male with a basal metabolic rate of around 2000 calories per day will get 275,000 units of antioxidants on an ORAC scale if he were to get all of his caloric needs met from plums only. If you were to eat a pound of boiled artichokes it will provide you with 42,000 ORAC units and 240 calories. One pound or 3 small red delicious apples will have around 19,000 ORAC units and 230 calories. We don't really need expensive "exotic" fruits and vegetables as a source of antioxidants. If you want to eat them that is great and we should eat as much as different varieties as we can but if you don't have money to waste on expensive produce regular apples will do. The real issue is that most people will eat low antioxidant vegetables and fruits and most of the calories will come from fat, sugar, meat, and junk. The small number of fruits and vegetables they will consume will likely be low on the antioxidant scale like bananas, cucumbers, iceberg lettuce, tomatoes, potatoes, peas and carrots and then will try to basically supplement with a couple of servings of some really exotic fruits for their antioxidant value. In the end, this approach will lead to very low antioxidant consumption. Instead of iceberg lettuce try to mix in some baby spinach and kale, some red beans and herbs, onions, garlic, and dill. Maybe some sprouts as well and some high nutrient dense whole food dressing instead of oil (an example will be some nut butter or tahini or avocado and lemon juice mix with some herbs). Just one teaspoon of an herb like rosemary on top of your salad can double its antioxidant content. Not everything has to be kale either. There is no need to deprive ourselves because we have to eat healthy all the time and force ourselves into food anxiety. If you like bananas eat bananas, the issue is that the average diet of average meat, sugar, and junk loving person is so bad and deprived of nutrients that some of the strategies I described here need to be implemented to help to balance the bad nutrient profile of the diet. If not, the end result can be chronic diseases and bad health. Some animal products on rare occasions are fine but if you are not vegan and I mean you don't eat whole food, plant based diet the reality is going to be that you probably have low antioxidant intake, low fiber intake, low mineral intake or unbalanced mineral profile of the diet with too little magnesium and iodine and selenium and so on. On top of that, it is likely that you will have an excessive amount of dietary cholesterol and saturated fat and on top of that, it is likely that you will be overexposed to environmental and dietary toxins. In this case, my advice is that if you cannot change your diet then you need to supplement. Even if you are vegan antioxidant optimization and supplementation will benefit you but more in line of prolonged longevity, boosted immune system, prevention of brain shrinkage, increased endurance, strength, overall wellbeing, and health. In non-vegan population supplementation with antioxidants will have longevity benefit too but the primary reason why they should do it is the prevention of chronic inflammatory conditions, cancer, cardiovascular, and other chronic diseases. Add more spice to a diet and just don't overdo on cinnamon and peppermint. Take turmeric as a supplement and amla and cloves and other herbs and spices. Take antioxidant rich essential oils. Drink cocoa and hibiscus and green tea. Increase your intake of antioxidant rich fruits and vegetables and add more variety to your diet. And of course, my recommendation for everyone is to take supplemental astaxanthin. One 12mg astaxanthin pill will be equivalent to taking 72g of vitamin C. That is 72,000 mg and unlike vitamin C it will not be excreted out. Astaxanthin is fat-soluble and it will bioaccumulate in tissue offering lasting protection.

After reading all about phytochemicals and antioxidants you might have a feeling that they are the same thing. Antioxidants are the most important phytochemicals for human health but actually, most of the phytochemicals have no antioxidant properties. Scientists estimate that there are more than 5,000 phytochemicals. There are tremendous amounts of ongoing research on them and in cases when a substance is proven to be beneficial that chemical can be patented and sold as medicine with a different name or used to make a supplement. There are 5,000 more potential drugs on the market. Some can be useful and are proven to be beneficial in different diseases and in general as health promoting substances. Some plants when tested have average antioxidant strength but are highly effective in fighting different types of diseases and they do this without any antioxidant properties. Depending on a disease or condition we want to prevent or help to heal we can review available science. For instance, because of all of the toxicity from the environment and bad diet cancer had become an epidemic and so are cardiovascular diseases. Prevention through diet is a reasonable option especially in cases of genetic predisposition and family history. If we look at the research into what plans can fight off cancer we will be surprised by the result because there are plants that are much more potent sources of antioxidants. This doesn't mean that antioxidants themselves do not fight cancer it just means that these plants have some unique phytochemicals that have biochemical reactions that will strongly suppress cancer cell's growth outside of any antioxidant activity. This is actually very good news because we can add them to our diet on top of any antioxidant rich food source we are already eating to have an additional synergistic effect. There are vegetables that are so good at fighting cancer that can rival any leading chemotherapy drug and at the same time target multiple different types of cancer cells. In this study (Antiproliferative and antioxidant activities of common vegetables: A comparative study. doi.org/10.1016/j.foodchem.2008.05.084) they tested 34 different vegetables on the proliferation of 8 different tumor cell lines in vitro. They used vegetable extract and drip them on different types of cancer cells to observe an effect on cancer growth. From all of the greens, spinach is one of the best, it is actually number two on the list in fighting against a pediatric brain tumor. Its suppressed brain tumor growth by nearly 100%. Only vegetable stronger in fighting brain tumor was beet. Spinach and beets are overall good at fighting all types of cancers. On another hand, there are vegetables that will still fight cancer cells but at levels of 10 to 40 percent suppression and are much weaker. Cucumbers, lettuce, tomatoes, potatoes, carrots, all the vegetables that people like to eat the most are very weak both in cancer prevention and in the antioxidant score. Most of the vegetables and fruit people commonly eat have no or very little effect. There was a vegetable that was so strong that the researchers were amazed. It blocked 100 percent of tumor cells growth in 7 out of 8 tumors tested. It was so strong that researchers wanted to test it on normal cells because they believed that there are some toxic phytochemicals in it that block any type of cells from multiplying not just cancer cells. They did test it on normal cells and cell growth was not affected at all. It is a vegetable that targets only cancer cells leaving normal cells alone and the only side effect is an increase in immune function, unlike regular chemotherapy. It was raw garlic extract. It was so strong that it rivaled leading chemotherapy drugs and it is selective, it goes out and attacks cancer cells leaving normal cells alone. What is unique about garlic? Nothing really, it is just more potent. The entire allium group of vegetables has the same or similar phytochemicals and will act the same way. Garlic is just the most potent vegetable from the entire group. It is an allium group of vegetables that is unique as a group because it has unique cancer-fighting phytochemicals. Garlic, onions, and leeks, in my opinion, should be added to salads on a daily bases just because of this study. It is an important finding. There are other benefits of garlic, some of them are proven in clinical trials but this is the most important find, maybe in the last couple of years. Allium family vegetables are potent chemotherapy drugs with no side effects. One clove of fresh garlic or some fresh onions or leeks is one good step in preserving health especially in people with a family history of cancer. For example, garlic is number one in breast cancer suppression. The problem is a strong smell that comes with garlic and that smell is exactly what makes it healthy. It is a natural insecticide that forms when something starts to chew on it. There is only one way to reap benefits from garlic and other allium family plants, and that is to eat them raw or to cut and crush them while raw and then eat them with no heating. Heating will destroy the cancer-fighting enzymes.

Other types of vegetables that are good in the fighting of cancer besides the allium group are the cruciferous vegetables. Kale, cabbage, red cabbage, cauliflower, broccoli, rutabaga, brussels sprouts. There is only one from the group that did not show any potential and that is bok choi. Odd one out. There are many phytochemicals in cruciferous vegetables from sulforaphane onward. Same as garlic they should be cut or chewed raw before cooking so that those insects fighting healthy beneficial chemicals like sulforaphane can form. I already wrote about the benefit of sulforaphane in a first book so I won't repeat it here. These are the two groups that are effective in cancer prevention and the rest of the vegetables are well below these two in effectiveness. These two groups plus spinach and beets are the vegetables to choose for our diet. There are not the antioxidant superstars but they don't have to be. The list of benefits that these two groups of vegetables bring to the table is long and serious. I won't analyze all of the clinical trials and health benefits I will only say this, if there is only one benefit from them and nothing else, if these vegetables are only good in cancer prevention and not one other thing, in my opinion, because of the levels of cancer in our society incorporating them into diet on a daily bases is reasonable choice just as a form of cancer prevention. The conclusion of the study was: "The extracts from cruciferous vegetables as well as those from vegetables of the genus Allium inhibited the proliferation of all tested cancer cell lines whereas extracts from vegetables most commonly consumed in Western countries were much less effective. The antiproliferative effect of vegetables was specific to cells of cancerous origin and was found to be largely independent of their antioxidant properties. These results thus indicate that vegetables have very different inhibitory activities towards cancer cells and that the inclusion of cruciferous and Allium vegetables in the diet is essential for effective dietary-based chemopreventive strategies."

On top of cruciferous vegetables and onions, there are some other food items that have specific phytochemicals that will have benefits like flaxseed. I recommend adding flaxseed in amounts of a couple of tablespoons in a week because of their high lignan content. There is a number of proven benefits of flaxseeds outside of its nutritious value and omega 3 content such as breast cancer prevention, lowering hypertension, helping weight loss but the main thing about them is that they are the richest source of lignans from all food. Flax may average a hundred times more lignans than other foods and lignans are actually the reason why they are good at preventing breast cancer in the first place. Lignans are one of the major classes of phytoestrogens, which are estrogen-like chemicals. The other classes of phytoestrogens are the isoflavones (from soy), and coumestans. The reason why they are good at balancing someone's hormone levels is that they are much weaker than human estradiol. Because they are not as potent as estrogen when they bind to the estrogen receptor, they are essentially blocking that receptor. They provide a weaker, cleaner estrogen to balance any deficit or surplus. They are estrogen receptor blockers. Tamoxifen (Nolvadex) that is prescribed for breast cancer does the exact same thing. Lignans in the females can help with hot flashes, balance hormones, and prevent breast cancer. In men, they can lower estrogen plus they can block the conversion of testosterone to DHT (dihydrotestosterone) and will help prevent prostate cancer, androgen pattern hair loss and at the same time will boost testosterone. Lowering DHT, lowering estrogen and boosting testosterone is every man's dream come true. Additionally, in both men and women, lignans inhibit the HSD enzyme, which helps reduce levels of the catabolic stress hormone, cortisol. It is the story the same as with soy. In normal amounts, lignans will help to balance the hormone levels meaning a couple of tablespoons during a week just don't overeat them in excessive amounts. Additionally for vegans, they are one if not the main source of omega 3 fatty acids. If you don't eat enough of omega 3 fatty acids, vegan or not, you might need to supplement with a marine algae source of DHA.

After reading all of this and on top of all of this still, there is a list of phytochemicals that can be beneficial and that are proven to be beneficial in clinical trials. I would not go any further into the analysis. Consider this book to be a starting point for you. Phytochemicals and especially antioxidants should be considered to be essential for life and we need to have awareness of them the same way that we have awareness for the necessity of vitamins. Because of the studies, there is no more debate in the scientific community in regard to their importance but there is the unwillingness to implement all of the knowledge into medical practice. There will be a day in the future when this would be common knowledge but until that time doctors will just prescribe pharmaceutical medicine as one and only solution to everything and will continue to do their job for the pharmaceutical industry. All health promoting advice will be condensed to basically losing weight and some essential diet correction like avoiding saturated fat and cholesterol and that will be it. Until things change you will be the one that has to acquire and also implement the knowledge that you will have to learn for yourself.

Minerals

"I had sinned against the wisdom of our creator, and received just punishment for it." - Justus von Liebig

How do you decide what to eat? Do you choose your food based on taste, price, current emotional state or this does not affect you at all? Maybe you choose what is quicker and does not require much time to be prepared, the so-called "fast food". In the developed world, the golden rule is that the time is money. The need for an individual to prepare food is just a waste of time, especially if you are overstressed and tired and have a lot of work to do. Therefore, fast food restaurants have become like gas stations: customers come in with their cars, food is pushed through the window and you drive off eating. The working man has become a machine in every possible way. Every day he needs to pour "fuel" and "oil" as quickly as possible in order to work. The problem with this type of behavior is that working man is a much more developed and complicated machine than manufacturing robot. Unlike a real machine that will immediately stop functioning in the event that it does not receive adequate fuel, the "human-machine" will not react in the same way. A human organism, since it is not a machine, in the case that it is not consuming the adequate amounts of nutrients from foods is still able to work for an extended period of time because the body is capable of taking the nutrients from its own reserves. It is a form of the loan and redistribution within the body itself. But if during that extended period, this "loan" does not compensate, the whole organism will eventually start to deteriorate and will gradually worsen until total collapse. Many of the diseases that have arisen over the last hundred years from the time of the Industrial Revolution are often the result of chronic malnutrition and disturbed metabolism. Most of the time these conditions will not be treated or will be misdiagnosed without anyone suspecting at them because these forms of diseases in most of the cases will not kill immediately but will create different kinds of conditions that are chronic and that will contribute to the overall state in which the body is in. This can then lead to more serious chronic conditions and real diseases. Believe it or not, this chronic malnutrition is the most widespread in the most economically developed countries and is present in most of the population. It is a result of the process that is known in nutrition as "empty calorie". There can be a lot of calories in the food that you eat and the food will be filled with fat and sugar but will have no minerals and at the same time will have a lot of toxins in it as well. Chronic malnutrition is the end result of the feverish effort of an organism to reach for the nutrients that cannot be found in food at all. Regardless of how much someone will eat and the quantity of the food that they will put into themselves, because there is nothing in that food except calories there can be a situation of morbid obesity and chronic malnutrition at the same time. And then doctors on top of that will advise the patients to lose weight, but will not advise the patients to increase the overall nutrient density of their diets. This can then lead to people going on the diets that are already chronically malnourished.

Unfortunately, today, people do not know that a group of doctors in the US Congress back in 1936 had already shown that it was "an alarming fact" that human food, fruits, vegetables and crops on millions of acres of land do not contain sufficient levels of all essential minerals, which will create chronic deficit and malnourishment no matter how much of the food people consume. This document (tabbed under number 264 at the 74th session of the Congress) was placed in an archive where until recently it was unavailable to the public. The important thing is that scientists were aware of the problem even back then. Eventually, it reached Congress. The title sheet says that it was presented by Mr. Fletcher. It is a reprint of Rex Beach's article about the work of Dr. Charles Northen, a physician who researched the soil replenishment to better nourish people and animals. He was based in Orlando, Florida, and could have been resident in Fletcher's constituency. It was presented by Mr. Fletcher and ordered to be printed by the United States Government Printing Office Washington. Here is what, among other things was found in the record:

Senate Document 264

74th Congress, 2nd Session, June 5, 1936

"Do you know that most of us today are suffering from certain dangerous diet deficiencies which cannot be remedied until depleted soils from which our food comes are brought into proper mineral balance?"

"The alarming fact is that foods (fruits, vegetables and grains) now being raised on millions of acres of land that no longer contain enough of certain minerals are starving us - no matter how much of them we eat. No man of today can eat enough fruits and vegetables to supply his system with the minerals he requires for perfect health because his stomach isn't big enough to hold them."

"The truth is that our foods vary enormously in value, and some of them aren't worth eating as food...Our physical well-being is more directly dependent upon the minerals we take into our systems than upon calories or vitamins or upon the precise proportions of starch, protein or carbohydrates we consume."

"This talk about minerals is novel and quite startling. In fact, a realization of the importance of minerals in food is so new that the textbooks on nutritional dietetics contain very little about it. Nevertheless, it is something that concerns all of us, and the further we delve into it the more startling it becomes."

"You'd think, wouldn't you, that a carrot is a carrot - that one is about as good as another as far as nourishment is concerned? But it isn't; one carrot may look and taste like another and yet be lacking in the particular mineral element which our system requires and which carrots are supposed to contain." "Laboratory test prove that the fruits, the vegetables, the grains, the eggs, and even the milk and the meats of today are not what they were a few generations ago (which doubtless explains why our forefathers thrived on a selection of foods that would starve us!)"

"No longer does a balanced and fully nourishing diet consist merely of so many calories or certain vitamins or fixed proportion of starches, proteins, and carbohydrates. We know that our diets must contain in addition something like a score of minerals salts."

"It is bad news to learn from our leading authorities that 99% of the American people are deficient in these minerals and that a marked deficiency in any one of the more important minerals actually results in disease. Any upset of the balance, any considerable lack of one or another element, however microscopic the body requirement may be, and we sicken, suffer, shorten our lives."

"We know that vitamins are complex chemical substances which are indispensable to nutrition and that each of them is of importance for the normal function of some special structure in the body. Disorder and disease result from any vitamin deficiency. It is not commonly realized, however, that vitamins control the body's appropriation of minerals, and in the absence of mineral's they have no function to perform. Lacking vitamins, the system can make some use of minerals, but lacking minerals, vitamins are useless."

"Certainly our physical well-being is more directly dependent upon the minerals we take into our systems than upon calories of vitamins or upon the precise proportions of starch, protein or carbohydrates we consume." "This discovery is one of the latest and most important contributions of science to the problem of human health."

".........this concludes Senate Document 264, 74th Congress, 2nd Session, June 5, 1936."

Dr. Northen further stated that some of the lands in the United States, even when not planted with crops at all, were still never balanced in terms of mineral composition. But in the end, no account was taken of this, and the use of both good and bad soil was done equally. Poor European immigrants encouraged to emigrate into the New World by the Catholic Church and overall bad conditions in Europe in the 18th century feverishly sought to grab as much land as possible especially near the rivers. All of the lands were "free" for them and they burned the forests and prairie in an effort to create fields for crop cultivation. However, due to the lack of minerals and already bad quality of the topsoil, many had poor yields and fattened and sick cattle. Those who were not able to leave the land would remain on it and still will be working on it trying to survive. They were using different methods to enrich the soil but that was not efficient in the grand scale of things and at that time the yields were much lower than they would be in the present-day industrial cultivation. Capitalism and the feverish pursuit of profit created a situation that by 1930 the land in Oklahoma, Texas, Nebraska, Kansas, and Iowa had already been completely eroded. The dry and failed crops grown on depleted soil is a situation that is visible immediately but this was not the case with humans and other animals. It took decades for the first symptoms to emerge in the general population. The land around the town of Midwest City, for example, was extremely poor with calcium. Three hundred children in the municipality were examined and close to 90% had poor teeth, 69% showed diseases, swollen gums, and diseased extremities. More than one-third had impaired vision, curved shoulders, and curved legs. Many disorders that are caused due to the lack of minerals in the diet have long been known to the scientists. It was nothing new even at the beginning of the 20th century. It was known that mice that lose their calcium in food are lagging behind in the development. Insufficient mineral input impairs their intelligence also. There was an experiment that showed that mice that had only this one mineral completely removed from the diet without any other restriction have difficulties to manage in the labyrinth. They had a hard time finding the way out. In addition, this can change their mood. They will become very agitated, turning themselves into cannibals. They will attack other mice in the community and will eat their flesh. If calcium is returned to the food, the group would become friendly and over time, everyone would again sleep peacefully in the crowd. Similarly, the different types of conditions will happen with every mineral element that plays a role in nutrition. Some deficiencies will affect behavior, some will affect the immune system and hormones and will cause pain and some deficiencies at least initially until they create some form of detectable damage will be completely symptom-free. The characteristic of the initial symptoms due to the different mineral deficiencies can vary. "Certainly our conditions are more dependent on the minerals we are taking than on calories or vitamins and regardless of the exact relationship of starch, protein, or carbohydrates we take," Dr. Northen suggested in 1936.

Dr. Harvey V. Weile was a doctor that was first appointed to the head of the US Chemical Bureau in 1906. This office later changed its name and is now called the Federal Food and Drug Administration (FDA). Without the approval of this agency, nothing can be introduced into the market. Chemical companies feverishly tried to get him thrown out and they had succeeded in 1912. Weile's policy even back then in 1912 was to feed people with food grown exclusively on naturally grown feeds, in order to contain all the necessary minerals and ingredients. This is nothing new. It is as old as human civilization. The science was well aware of this more than 100 years ago. But the resilience of large-scale capital was huge. His memoirs and documents demonstrating his struggle for healthy nutrition were published in the book in 1930 after having faced the heavy obstruction of the publisher. Today, most of these books have been removed from all US libraries or destroyed. But the real "destructive bomb" for human health is actually a "cure" against land depletion. These are now irreplaceable artificial fertilizers.

The artificial fertilizer inventor is the celebrated German chemist Justus von Liebig (1803-1873). In 1831 he became a real "chemical superstar" after discovering chloral and chloroform (used by doctors as a narcotic). He later received the title of "father" of organic chemistry. Liebig has been researching various chemical processes in the physiology of animals and chemical and physical laws in the maintenance of life and health and studied the products of tissue decomposition. He classified various diets in accordance with the special functions and needs in every animal species and also did a nutritional analysis. Similar to nutritional specialists of today but he also did experiments in agricultural production with a goal to increase farming effectiveness and profit. And, contrary to many medical thoughts of that time, he thought that the body's heat was the result of the combustion and oxidation in the body itself. The result of his studies was the preparation of food for children from meat extracts. When he began to study the physiology of plants, he specifically devoted himself to agriculture that he considered being the basis of every trade and industry. Nonetheless, improvements in the field of agriculture cannot be rationally applied without understanding certain chemical principles that would be more effective. You may not know this, but this is a typical modern scientific way of perceiving the world, which does not mean that Liebig was aware of it. Scientists believe that nature is not efficient enough and that a man can create much better (and more profitable, of course) solutions. Thus, in 1840, Liebig in his book "Organic chemistry in its applications to agriculture and physiology" dismissed the old notion that plants draw their nutrient ingredients from humus, but thought they were taking carbon and nitrogen from carbon dioxide and ammonia present in the atmosphere, and then these ingredients will be returned to the atmosphere by the process of rotting and fermentation, which he considered an essential chemical process in nature while potash (potassium carbonate), sodium carbonate, lime, sulfur, phosphorus, etc. ... come from the soil. Carbon dioxide and ammonia do not cause depletion of the soil, but the mineral ingredients are limited because the soil cannot afford their unlimited quantities. Thus, according to Liebig, the main concern of the farmer was to restore the soil with only those minerals that are known to play a role in the crop production and which they use in their growth. These are the minerals that are found in the ash of crops after its incineration. His theory consequently showed that there was a "law of minimum" for fertilizing crops and he considered that nitrogen, phosphorus, and potassium could increase crop production proportionally. Crops could be fed synthetically with those minerals. After several years of promoting this theory, it was accepted and implemented in practice and he prepared artificial fertilizers containing artificially produced minerals together with small amounts of ammonia salts. The fertilized yields were really huge, with only three minerals. Nitrogen, phosphorus, and potassium proved that they are able to make synthetic soil "enough" to stimulate the growth of fruits and vegetables. The only problem is that all of the fruits and vegetables were in a serious failure of all other minerals that were naturally found in the soil, while some crops did not contain anything at all. And without all of the necessary minerals, vitamins cannot be transported and many other functions of the human body would fail also. The human organism has a more complex structure than one of the plants and needs a different and more complex profile of minerals. But at that time that idea didn't cross his mind. Later analyzing these imperfect fruits, Liebig officially renounced his theories and rejected the idea of a possible synthetic feeding of crops:

"I had sinned against the wisdom of our creator and received just punishment for it. I wanted to improve his handiwork, and in my blindness, I believed that in this wonderful chain of laws, which ties life to the surface of the earth and always keeps it rejuvenated, there might be a link missing that had to be replaced by me--this week, powerless nothing. The law, to which my research on the topsoil led me, states, 'On the outer crust of the earth, under the influence of the sun, organic life shall develop', and so, the great master and builder gave the fragments of the earth the ability to attract and hold all these elements necessary to feed plants and further serve animals, like a magnet attracts and holds iron particles, so as no piece to be lost. Our master enclosed a second law unto this one, through which the plant bearing earth becomes an enormous cleansing apparatus for the water. Through this particular ability, the earth removes from the water all substances harmful to humans and animals--all products of decay and putrefaction, of perished plant and animal generations. What might justify my actions is the circumstance, that a man is the product of his time, and he is only able to escape the commonly accepted views if a violent pressure urges him to muster all his strength to struggle free of these chains of error. The opinion, that plants draw their food from a solution that is formed in the soil through rainwater, was everyone's belief. It was engraved into my mind. This opinion was wrong and the source of my foolish behavior. When a chemist makes a mistake in rating agricultural fertilizers, don't be too critical of his errors, because he has had to base his conclusions upon facts which he can't know from his own experience, but rather, has to take from agricultural texts as true and reliable. After I learned the reason why my fertilizers weren't effective in the proper way, I was like a person that received a new life. For along with that, all processes of tillage were now explained as to their natural laws. Now that this principle is known and clear to all eyes, the only thing that remains is the astonishment of why it hadn't been discovered a long time ago. The human spirit, however, is a strange thing. Whatever does not suit him in his scope of thought, it does not exist for him."

For every scientist to this day, nature is flawed and can and will be "improved" if we can use the laws of biology and physics to our advantage. People have long known a number of ways to slow down the process of mineral depletion of the soil: green manure (plant residues from crops protecting against wind erosion, retaining moisture and adding nitrogen to the soil), stacking plants and animal waste to land, the use of guan (a bird-rich fertilizer rich in nitrogen), and so on. Even the Bible wrote that every seven years the soil must be left to rest. Nevertheless, scientific philosophy prevailed. The essence of our reality is the fact that civilization we know and live in today is entirely based on scientific philosophy and represents the form of scientific existentialism as a religion. This belief is that man is God on Earth who has the power to create (thought numerous technical achievements) and to overlay what is naturally created. The consequences are as follows: human habitat as well as modern philosophy are so abridged and separated from natural ("divine laws") that today's urban people can hardly accept life without civilization. Survival in nature has become a big problem for an urban man of today - he is dependent on technology, a system that provides it and money. If there is some emergency, or war, or new ice age, or global warming, or any form of disaster it would create the starvation of most of the global population in a very short period. Pentagon actually did social and military analyses of this. The time period needed is two weeks. It is two weeks that is needed to deplete food stores in cities around the world and millions of people would be starved of hunger. Food is transported into cities and if something collapses the economy there is no more transportation of food and self-sufficiency. Life in the city actually had already became organized and controlled as a labor camp. Life without cars and TVs for many people has long since become unimaginable. Consequently, there was a complete adaptation to an unnatural way of life, as the man was designed by man, and not by nature. Consequences of this essential change of the world must logically manifest somewhere, and that is the tribute that is already paid in the most economically developed societies: people can no longer live without drugs and live shorter with increasing consumption of food that they cannot produce for themselves and are depended on large scale monoculture production with GMO's grown on a land depleted off all minerals. Artificial fertilizers undoubtedly brought bigger crops, higher yields, and better earnings. Justus von Liebig is deliberately forgotten (he is not taught in schools), and the false fertilizers he renounced were put into circulation. Thus many farmers propagated by bad teachings and propaganda reoriented themselves from natural to artificial fertilizers. Knowledge about the true fertilization of the land that was passed for thousands of years from one generation to another was abended overnight. Synthetic fertilizers are manmade inorganic compounds - usually derived from by-products of the petroleum industry. Examples are superphosphate, ammonium phosphate, ammonium nitrate, and potassium sulfate. The superstar product of the new agricultural philosophy is superphosphate, which many call the mother of all false fertilizers. The mineral nutritional deficit has thus become a common phenomenon in the most economically developed world.

And what will you do now when you read this? You think you can go to the pharmacy and look for minerals in the pills, don't you? A typical "scientific" mindset, of course. You started to believe that a man can ruin everything he can and then just have a simple fix because man is the same as God the Creator. Just need the money and a good pharmacy, right? Well, not so quickly. Nature did not invent a mineral tablet. All essential minerals we need cannot be created unless they are created by the same force that created the man himself. And man did not create himself. Nature did.

Metal inorganic minerals come from different types of stones like limestone (calcium carbonate), chemicals and petroleum industry and clay. Mineral extracts for human consumption are made from these types of inorganic materials. Most of these minerals have a toxic effect on the body. The first problem is in their absorption. Some animals can easily absorb inorganic minerals, but for the human body, it is a difficult process because we have the acidity of pH4 with food in our stomach and that is not enough to ionize these metallic minerals. If for example, dog eats a metal penny, it would be eventually almost completely dissolved the same as bones because a dog is a carnivore and like other carnivores have the acidity of pH 1 with food in the stomach. If we consume inorganic metals they need to be destroyed by acid into their monoatomic form to be used correctly in the body. The reason is the size of the mineral compared to the size of the cell. Are you able to swallow the whole loaf of bread? No, but you will chew and cut the loaf with the knife. The cells in our bodies do not have a "knife".

There is a big difference between inorganic and organic minerals. Realistically, minerals are just inorganic metals, so it makes no difference where you get them. The most important factor when we talk about organic vs. inorganic minerals is not composition, it is the same metal, but it is the size and the form they are in. If the size of minerals is not small enough for us to use them in biological functions we call them inorganic, not because they are some other molecular substance but just because the size of the molecule is too big. They are small but not small enough, at least not small enough to be used as an organic form of minerals. There is only one way that the human digestive system can break down larger tightly bound minerals into usable ions, and that is with the stomach acid. The food transit time through the stomach is about one hour. If the inorganic mineral ion is not ionized during this small amount of time and mineral moves from the high acid environment of the stomach no further beneficial breakdown will take place in the small intestines. All further break down ceases. If the inorganic mineral compound is already relatively small like from deep spring water, it might get degraded to smaller monoatomic scale particles by the acid in the stomach and be bioavailable. Once minerals left the acidic environment of the stomach the remainder of the non-ionized minerals are of no use for us and are in no way available to do any biological functions inside our body except negative ones. Usually, they will just pass through our GI tract unusable. But If you ingest big chunks of metals called inorganic minerals they might end up in the bloodstream in small quantities. However, they can pass into the bloodstream in large quantities if you have leaky gut or inflammation in the intestines. They will not be small enough to integrate into cells or do any other biological function and will create deposits in the body if the body does not remove them out in time.

When vitamin-mineral tablets, metallic minerals, and minerals or their salts are taken, the body absorbs only 8 to 12%, into the bloodstream while the rest simply passes through the intestines. Even what is absorbed is not really useable because it is still in inorganic form. In order to solve this problem, which was apparently known to them, pharmacists invented the so-called "chelated minerals" in the seventies: they were wrapped in amino acids and other substances to help the body to absorb them. Minerals through human evolution were abundant and protein was scarce. So body adapted mechanism to absorb minerals only through diffusion. What that means is that the body will do absolutely nothing to absorb minerals and will only let some of them pass through the intestinal lining by themselves. There is an electrical charge in the ionic organic minerals that will attract them like a magnet to the intestinal lining and then they will pass into the bloodstream. Amino acids (protein) on the other hand are absorbed proactively. Our bodies adapted mechanisms to actively absorb them because there was scarcity in normal evolutionary conditioning. Consequently, what scientists working for the Big Pharma theorized is that if they bound amino acids to the inorganic minerals chemically, the body will actively absorb that amino acid and as a consequence will also pull this inorganic form of metallic mineral with it. Inorganic minerals have a different charge then organic ions and are repelled by the charge of the intestinal lining if the lining is healthy and there is no inflammation in the gut. It is a form of evolutionary protective mechanism against inorganic metallic mineral absorption. But when you "chelate them" with amino acids or some other substances, then it is a different story. This contributed to their absorption rate to rise up to 50%.

So how does a human organism take minerals at all, you're wondering? Simply - all minerals in fruits and vegetables are colloidal (organic). The colloid means a substance that exists in extremely fine particles that are present in the media of various materials. The colloid state is the state of the solution (minerals or some other substances) where the molecules of that substance form soluble particles. A plant takes the artificial, inorganic minerals from the soil where it is growing that are big chunks of metal if you like that analogy. When plants take up inorganic minerals from the ground by the roots then they synthesize them, or if you like break them down into a molecular size and form that is small enough to do regular biological functions in the living matter. There are also microbes in the soil that will do this just by themselves and will help the plant root system to absorb all of the minerals plant needs. S. Vojutsky wrote in 1975 the classic text about colloidal chemistry. According to him, colloidal systems must have three basic characteristics:

1. Must be diverse (to contain different ingredients which are not similar)

2. Must be multiphase (e.g. solid-liquid, etc.)

3. particles must be insoluble in solution.

It is precisely the colloids of minerals in plants that remain heterogeneous, multifaceted and insoluble in varying concentrations. The plants convert metallic minerals from the soil into this form through photosynthesis and they become part of the plant. Colloidal minerals compared to those of shellfish is as if you were to compare the eating of veal with cartilage. Dogs can eat cartilage and bones, but humans cannot. Each particle of colloidal minerals is hundreds of times smaller than inorganic mineral particles. Plant colloids are the smallest particles of matter that can be divided but still have all of their features. The blood cell is 7 microns (6 - 8 μm). The colloidal particle is 0.01 micron or less and this is a 700th part of the size of the blood cell. And this is the right measure for the size of the bite the cell can swallow. All particles of colloidal minerals are also naturally negatively charged which attracts them to the walls of the intestinal lining that have a natural positive charge, like an iron magnet. Due to this negative charge and low weight, they remain floating in the solution and do not bound together to form a solid-state. Inorganic minerals have a positive charge and are not intended to be absorbed in the human organism. Even if you were to eat the soil itself you would not be able to absorb them. The human organism is not intended to absorb non-organic matter. In addition, many can be toxic if they accumulate in the tissue. For example, if you swallow inorganic form of arsenic, lead, alumina and other minerals that are considered toxic you can kill yourself. Dr. Kerry Rims, a renowned biochemist and biophysicist, discovered that colloids can be so small that they can pass through the glass. These tiny particles have a small "solar system" around them so that around one particle can circle more than a few of the different minerals. Basically, they pull each other. Dr. Rhymes discovered that a human body requires 84 of the 106 known elements to be healthy. This is far more than it is officially proclaimed. In one of the abandoned mines in Utah (USA), one local ranger reportedly discovered in 1925 large amounts of deposited fossils containing preserved minerals in a colloidal state, which are today sold on the market as a supplement. They have found over 65 different minerals and traces of minerals in those deposited fossils. That means that fossils that where once living creatures had 65 different colloidal minerals doing something in their body. We don't know and do not have science for all minerals that are biologically active. We have research in calcium, magnesium, potassium and so on but not for all of 65 different minerals that are proven to have some biochemical reactions in the body that are not toxic.

Thus, only plants can take inorganic ingredients from the soil and make from them the living organic matter that we eat. The animals are there to consume them only and don't produce anything. Animals just accumulate living matter and energy from the plants. Animals are uses and only users. Plants are the only ones that can create new organic matter using solar energy. It is clear that nature is created in the following order and the hierarchy that begins on soil: soil, plants, animals, and humans. Science teaches us the opposite: people, animals, plants. Sick soil means sick plants, sick animals, sick people. You cannot fix the state of malnutrition just by using patented drugs.

Suppose that some organism is, for instance, deficient with copper. Copper is used for radio frequency (RF) shielding because it absorbs radio and electromagnetic waves. When it comes to blocking EMF radiation, you'll often see copper used as a wire mesh, which will completely block both radio and microwave radiation. Consequently, it is the only metal that is used in neurons in the brain to create the electric discharge. For coppering myelin coating in the nerve cells, copper is needed as a good conductor. If you are deficient in the copper, for example, your brain will have difficulties especially in the part of myelin formation (Myelin and traumatic brain injury: The copper deficiency hypothesis. doi.org/10.1016/j.mehy.2013.09.011). The most common cause of copper deficiency is a gastrointestinal surgery, such as gastric bypass surgery, due to malabsorption of copper, or zinc toxicity. This is just copper. How about 64 other minerals that we need and don't get in our modern diet?

To exactly understand what is going on in medicine and nutrition I will use another field of medicine as a comparison. In the agricultural industry and farming operations, there is no such thing as health insurance. There is no profit to be made out of sick animals, quite the opposite. In human medicine, the interest is to use the most expensive treatments that we can find to make the biggest profit we can without killing the patient for an extended period of time. In the agricultural industry, it is completely the opposite. When dealing with domesticated animals, the interest is to use the most cost-effective treatments and to heal the animals as much as possible without any expensive drugs or treatments because that will decrease our profit when we want to sell that meat or milk. That is why overuse of antibiotics is implemented and many other practices that are cost-effective. But what about nutrition deficiencies? Animal feed is also grown on depleted soil. There is a good book on the subject from doctor Joel Wallach named "Dead Doctors Don't Lie." He had done a lot of work with livestock and had a degree in agriculture and then went to veterinary school. As a veterinary student, he learned the most cost-effective ways to heal diseases in animals with nutrition unlike in medical schools. Nutrition is the most cost-effective way to heal the animals and that is what the students are learning. Animals don't have Medicare. If you want to be a farmer then you must learn how to do things efficiently with just feed and nutrition. After spending two years in Africa working with large animals he was asked to come to the Saint Louis Zoo to work on a special project. They received a 7.5 million dollars grant from the National Institute for Health to do autopsies of animals that have died there in the zoo from natural causes. Usually, animals just die without cancer or diabetes or heart disease. Animals usually when they are in the zoo die from aging. In the wild, they typically die from starvation or predation or disease. To be precise, veterinarians use to think that in the zoo animals die from natural causes, but they were wrong. Dr. Wallach did autopsies in the Brookfield Zoo in Chicago, LA Zoo, National Zoo, Bronx Zoo in New York and others. They also wanted to find what species of animals are sensitive to what kinds of toxins or pollution. Animals are exposed in much higher levels to all of the toxins in the human environment then they would be exposed in nature. In the next 12 years, he performed 17,500 autopsies on 454 different species of animals. That is a large and significant number and this is plenty of data to analyze. Now in his own words and I am not saying that this is correct but what he found was that every single case of death of natural causes in these animals was some form of nutritional deficiency. That was challenging for him to explain and was also very interesting at the same time that every single animal species in captivity dies from a nutritional deficiency, not aging. This could be scientifically documented in the autopsies and it was not just an opinion. He published 75 scientific articles as a consequence of this research and also eight multi-author textbooks and so on but people just didn't want to listen. Nobody seemed to care. He was going from newspapers to magazines to TV networks. Nobody cared back in the 60s about nutrition. Actually, nobody was allowed to care in human medicine about nutrition because that would be a direct opposite of the medical industry line of conducting business. As long as it used for animals it is ok. As soon as somebody had a stupid idea to talk about nutrition in human society it was suppressed. After all of this, and stable and good job with a good salary, he was angry and irritated, and decided he is going to go to school again to become a regular physician. He wanted to implement everything he learned from all of the animal autopsies in his veterinary practice to healing human patients and wanted to prove his work. Then he worked 12 years in Portland Oregon in general practice and tested all of his theses. He also had a thesis that real genetic potential for the human lifespan is between 120 and 140 years. This can sound strange to you but actually, there are cases of people, documented cases of people, living more than this. The longest living person was one Chinese man dr. Li (Li Ching-Yuen) that lived 256 years. He was a doctor of Chinese natural medicine, not a Western medicine doctor. He was born in 1677, and 150 years later he was given a certificate by in that time the Chinese Imperial Government for being 150 years old. 50 years later the same Imperial Government gave him a second certificate. Some documents credit him with 24 marriages more than 180 descendants in 11 generations in the time of his death. And no it is not a mistake or a hoax it is well documented. In 1749, at 72 years of age, he joined the Chinese Imperial Government army of Yeuh Jong Chyi, provincial Commander-in-Chief, as a tactical advisor and as a teacher of martial arts and this is something we can check in historical records. Li avoided smoking or drinking liquor, he had a vegetarian diet and he was known to eat a lot of different kinds of berries on a daily basis that he was collecting from nature and had cultivated goji berry plants himself. He frequently had goji berry tea as well. When he died back in 1933 the London Times wrote an article about his death. Corruption in the medical industry is what is trying to keep this information out of public awareness. Today there are 5 cultures that have a lifespan that averages above 100 years of age disease-free. From famous Hunza people to Tibetans in Western China who were popularized in 1934 by James Hilton that wrote a book named "The Lost Horizon". It was a Pulitzer Prize-winning book. The average lifespan in Western civilization is around 75 with different chronic diseases most of that life. The average lifespan of a doctor is even considerably shorter than the national average and they blame that fact on stress.

To have all of the nutrients you need for survival you will have to consume adequate amounts of 60 minerals, in the fossil record, there are 65 minerals so the real number will be from 60 to 65 different organic colloidal minerals. Then 16 vitamins. Then you need 12 essential amino acids that you already probably have too much of. Then you need the energy in the form of sugar or oil. Then you will need 3 essential fatty acids. On top of that, you will need an adequate amount of fiber for the healthy microbiome in the gut and detoxification. Then more than 20,000 units of different types of antioxidants in a day. Then you will need all of the different phytochemicals that are known to have biochemical reactions in the body. Now, this is a substantial list. And no you don't need cholesterol, our liver produces that substance in an adequate amount. For us, it is not a nutrient. It is an anti-nutrient that creates arteriosclerosis and plaque. So, how much nutrients do you think you can get with food that is grown on depleted soil? Or how much of nutrients you think you will consume in animal products in animals that are fed with the food that is grown on mineral-depleted soil? When we look at charts of different food items it is all just a scam. I want to repeat this. When we look at the charts of nutritional content meaning how much minerals are in the different vegetables it is irrelevant and it is just a scam. Why? Because there are no minerals in vegetables that are grown in mineral-depleted soil. These charts are made from analyzing healthy organically grown plants. That is not a food item that you will find in a store. Even organic food today is of significantly lesser quality then what the real foods used to be. Only in plant sources, like for example nuts, would be a good example, you will have the high nutritional values you can read in the nutrition charts. Why nuts? Because it takes 10 years for a walnut tree to grow to produce a nut. And the walnut tree is big, and has a big root system that grows deep into the soil that has not been eroded too much and depleted. Eating plants that are grown in one season and then harvested like corn, rice, grains, beans, potatoes, and other vegetables is useless. Their real nutritional value is zero. Let me repeat this again. The real nutritional value is zero. These vegetables are mineral depleted and grown on commercial land year, after year, after year, for hundreds of years by now. Plants can be grown even hydroponically on sponges and UV lamps. There is no difference between a sponge that is infused with artificial fertilizer and water and the land that is eroded and mineral depleted. Hydroponically grown tomatoes might look like real tomatoes but it is just an illusion. There are no minerals in them. There will be a lot of vitamins and lycopene and other antioxidants and phytochemicals in them that plant can produce just by itself, but there will be no minerals in them. There is no plant in existence that can create atomic molecules like metals out of thin air. There must be different types of minerals that are present in the soil, all 65 of them so that plant can pick them up from the soil and then convert them to colloidal form so that when we eat that tomato it will have them all. If you don't consume all of those minerals in adequate amounts in some prolonged-time period, you will develop a nutritional disease. The medical profession is so busy saving people with chemotherapy and patented medicine that somehow they forget to educate people about nutritional density and to test people for different forms of deficiencies. They don't even want to recognize the fact that the human body needs 65 minerals to function properly and don't even want to recognize the fact that antioxidants and phytochemicals are essential for human life as well. They don't even want to recognize the fact that fiber is an essential nutrient. Only vitamins and protein end essential amino acids and essential oils are recognized as essential. Everything else is not. Some smaller number of minerals are recognized as essential, basically only the main ones while the rest of them is just ignored as rare earth minerals that are not important. They don't even know or want to investigate in the studies what all of this trace and rare earth minerals do in the body. There is some amount of research but that is nothing compared with the research done for patented medicine and chemotherapy and all other things that are going to be in the line of conducting business. Most of that money we give to medical business is going to Big Pharma and doctors Mercedes and mortgage payments and holiday. We are paying them to basically waste our own money because of our own ignorance. Most of the population, I will say more than 99% never heard anything about this. Most of the population has no idea that there is something like minerals or understand that land, where the crops are grown, is not some dirt that has no meaning to our lives but actually that dirt is one and the same thing as our intestinal lining. That soil composition and everything that is in there good or bad is going directly to your bloodstream and if the soil is depleted the plant will be depleted and then your body will be empty as well. Most people just know about calcium because that is what propaganda is teaching so that they will consume dairy products, or iron because of anemia so that they will consume a lot of meat and that is it. What does the selenium do in our body? How about iodine? How about chromium? Medical care is not free. It is just a propaganda design for you to believe that it is free. It is one of the most expensive evil industries. I have personally worked in the medical college and have direct personal perspective about the psychological profile of people going to the medical schools. There are there to make money. There are investing in their future career. Medicine is filled with intelligent and ambitious individuals eager to have six-figure salaries. No one is going to invest that much of his or her money, time and effort just to help people. They have student debts and loans and mortgages and a license that can be annulled. That is the reality. They will give Hippocratic oath but that is just propaganda. If we use human type medicine to treat livestock your hamburger will cost 300 dollars. On another hand if we use the same model that is used in veterinary medicine your average health insurance for a family of 4 will be 10 to 20 dollars a month. That is why nobody is thought nutrition in medical schools. That is why nobody is talking about nutrition in TV programs or any mainstream media. Who is going to believe me instead of a certified specialist with different titles giving him advice on what to do or what pills or surgery to have?

For example, they have known more than 50 years ago that ulcers in pigs are caused not by stress but by Helicobacter pylori so with a trace mineral called bismuth they were able to treat and cure stomach ulcers in pigs without surgery so that your meat is economically sustainable. It cost 5 dollars to cure one pig of stomach ulcers. If you have an ulcer a teaspoon of Pepto-Bismol is all you need.

If they wanted to prevent kidney stones in livestock they gave them calcium, magnesium, and boron and were considering kidney stone as a calcium deficiency disease because the body will pull out excessive amount of calcium from the bones and some of it will end up in the kidneys or if animals have magnesium deficiency calcium enzymes won't work so calcium will stay in the bloodstream causing kidney stones and calcium deposits. That was their line of reasoning and they did manage to cure kidney stones with the addition of mineral supplements. If cattle get kidney stones, they die. It is called a water belly. A farmer will have a problem if an animal dies before he is able to send it to the market so in veterinary medicine they learned how to prevent this more than 50 years ago by increasing calcium and magnesium and boron in the diet. It was only in 1995 that regular medicine acknowledged this. Here is a part of this study (Calcium intake and urinary stone disease doi: 10.3978/j.issn.2223-4683.2014.06.05): "For many years patients were advised to decrease their calcium intake in an attempt to limit the hypercalciuria (high blood levels of calcium) as dietary calcium restriction was one of the mainstays of therapy for prevention of stone recurrence. Large, prospective observational studies were the first to demonstrate the potential risks of low calcium intake. Using data from more than 45,000 men in the Health Professionals Follow-up Study, Curhan et al. were the first to demonstrate in their 1993 article that low dietary calcium intake potentially increased the risk of stones by more than 51% compared to men with the highest dietary calcium intake. These findings were later confirmed with a similar effect in both younger and older women in the Nurses Health Studies II and I respectively, and more recently in the women in the observational arm of the Women's Health Initiative. Dietary calcium intake is likely a protective factor against the stone formation and this is likely the case whether dietary calcium comes from dairy or non-dairy sources."

Calcium is a well-known mineral in the general public and there is not much to say about it. Green leafy vegetables have enough bioavailable calcium and there is no osteoporosis in rural parts of the world that are poor and undeveloped and lactose intolerant. For example, African woman do not get osteoporosis on 300mg of calcium a day. African blacks are 98 percent lactose intolerant. Most of us have enough calcium and in some cases, the excessive amount of calcium because of our shift in the diet. Osteoporosis is not usually caused by calcium deficiency. There is truth however in the fact that if you are vegan and don't consume dairy then calcium deficiency might pose a problem if you don't eat enough of calcium-rich organically grown produce. It is not a vegan diet that will cause it and people need to understand this. In regular commercial products levels of calcium can be zero because of the soil depletion. But what about all other minerals that are not so well known?

For example, what can just one mineral deficiency like copper cause? Aneurysms besides brain damage are one more thing that can be caused by copper deficiency. In one case in 1957 around 250,000 turkeys had died and were autopsied. More than half of the entire population on one big industrial farm had died in a period of 13 weeks. The farmer didn't know what is wrong so doctor Joel Wallach and his team were sent to investigate. What they found out was that all of them, every single one turkey had died from a ruptured aortic aneurysm. So they doubled the amount of copper in the food pallets, in that time that was the treatment for an aneurysm in animals because usually, they do not have arteriosclerotic plaque, so the only possible cause can be a copper deficiency. In the next year, the same farm didn't lose one single turkey. Later the same experiment had been performed on mice and rabbits and other species and it was always the same. In human's stroke is usually a consequence of bad diet same as heart disease but in animals, it is usually because of mineral deficiencies. This, however, doesn't mean that if you have a copper deficiency that this cannot happen in you as well. Copper plays a role in the functioning of elastic fibers in blood vessels. Without copper, the blood vessels lose their elasticity and will become brittle. So, for example, chronic copper deficiency can cause a stroke or varicose veins. It can also cause gray hair independently from stress or aging.

Selenium deficiency has been associated with infertility, cardiovascular disease, myodegenerative diseases, and cognitive decline. In Europe entire soil everywhere is severely selenium deficient. In the US most of the soil that is used for crops, even organic produce is also selenium deficient. Cardiomyopathy (a weakened heart muscle) for example (Keshan disease) is just selenium deficiency. An individual with Keshan disease will have an abnormally large heart. It can cause white muscle disease or stiff lam disease in animals and because of it today any farmer can go to the store and get selenium pallets. Cardiomyopathy can be prevented with adequate selenium intake. At least this form of it like Keshan disease. In regular medicine when asked the answer will be that in many cases, the cause of cardiomyopathy isn't known. That is not complete truth and especially is hard for them to explain the cases when the disease occurs in children. Some other types are called "unclassified cardiomyopathy" and so on and this is regular medical science. They will treat this disease with medications, surgery and different forms of implanted devices to correct arrhythmias. Cardiomyopathy was firstly associated with selenium deficiency in China in modern medicine but in veterinary medicine, they have known about it for 50 years. Another cause of cardiomyopathy can be one type of virus named the Coxsackie virus. If you are already selenium deficient and then get infected by the virus that attacks heart muscle, it is a bad combination. The heart can be damaged also by coronary heart disease and weakened by some other diseases and conditions as well, but these are different diseases. Have you ever seen some professional athletes like soccer players that are considered to be perfectly healthy that just drop dead on the field from arrhythmias like Endurance Indahor from Sudan or Piermario Morosini from Italy? For instance, a soccer player named Serginhno from Brazil was just standing and in the next 10 seconds, he was on the ground dead from sudden cardiac death. These are young athletes that have constant medical testing. Some of these cases may be due to the hypertrophic cardiomyopathy (a portion of the heart becomes thickened) that can be genetic but some of them are just selenium deficiency that caused the cardiomyopathy. These are professional athletes and would know if they had any hypertrophic thickening of the heart. What about just regular people with no heart disease that just drop dead in the middle of the street from a cardiomyopathy heart attack. That is cardiomyopathy or severe selenium deficiency if you don't have the hypertrophic thickening of the heart or any other form of a heart condition. Moderate deficiency is linked to prostate cancer, infertility in men, muscle weakness, depressed mood, anxiety, and neurological diseases. Kashin-Beck disease that creates deformity of bones, cartilage, and joints especially in children 5 to 13 years of age that is present in parts of, China, Tibet, North Korea, and Siberia is caused by selenium deficiency. Heart transplant for cardiomyopathy patients cost is 750,000 dollars. The heart is free and the blood is free from good people that are donors. Even if the individual patients are able to pay for this insane price, availability is extremely limited. More than 116,000 Americans are waiting to receive a transplant, and about 20 die each day during the wait. Maybe it would be cost-effective if people just learn more about their diet. Still don't believe me, ok read this then (Fulminant heart failure due to selenium deficiency cardiomyopathy (Keshan disease). Med Sci Law. 2002 Jan;42(1):10-3) or this (A Rare Cause of Cardiomyopathy: A Case of Selenium Deficiency Causing Severe Cardiomyopathy that Improved on Supplementation doi: 10.7759/cureus.1627). The conclusion of the second study was: "Patients with malnutrition and signs of heart failure should be screened for a deficiency in micronutrients such as Se, as cardiomyopathy may be reversible with Se supplementation." How many people eat Brazil nuts? How many people eat artificial fertilizer hydroponically grown mineral depleted food? In the U.S. the situation is not as bad as in Europe because selenium is given to the animals as a supplement in the feed. Furthermore, selenium concentration in soil has a lesser effect on selenium levels in animal products than in plant-based foods because animals maintain predictable tissue concentrations of selenium through homeostatic mechanisms. Animals will not excrete selenium because it is already needed so any amount they get will be incorporated into the cells and saved. But for vegans and vegetarian's selenium deficiency is a concern. The lowest selenium intakes in the world are in certain parts of China where large sections of the population have a mostly vegetarian diet and soil selenium levels are very low. Average selenium intake is also low in some European countries, especially among populations consuming vegan diets. So if you are vegan and you don't eat organic or for that matter even do my advice will be to add Brazil nuts and other selenium-rich food. Land in South America is rich in selenium and roots of the Brazil nut tree are deep so it should have the level of selenium in it that we can see in the charts. Brazil nuts contain very high amounts of selenium (68-91 mcg per nut) and could even cause selenium toxicity if consumed regularly. Acute selenium toxicity can cause a lot of issues and can actually be lethal as well with kidney failure and cardiac failure. Light acute toxicity can give you muscle tenderness, gastrointestinal and neurological symptoms, hair loss, acute respiratory distress syndrome, facial flushing, tremors, and lightheadedness. Therefore, don't overdo with supplemental selenium and don't eat Brazil nuts every day as a snack. They can be toxic. Maybe just one a day maximum. Or even one in a couple of days if you are not vegan.

So what happens when you are deficient, how would you know if you are lacking some minerals in the first place? If we are lacking in regular calories we will feel hungry but how could we know if we are lacking in some nutrients except to do some laboratory test? In animals, there is a phenomenon known as pica. Pica is the desire to eat unusual substances that possess little or no nutritional value to the animal such as dirt or wood or bone. Farmers know about this and will give cattle some minerals or they might chew on feed bunk. Because cattle lose a lot of minerals in constant milking it is not uncommon to see them chewing almost everything from bone to the bark. There is still the lacking of consensus, is this real physiological craving as a result of for example calcium deficiency, or it is something animals do out of some instinctive trigger. In humans, pregnant women are notorious for pica. They will have cravings for all sorts of different food items, not just pickles. A growing baby will pull a lot of minerals from the mother's body and that might be a cause of this. Lacking minerals can be manifested as a craving for salt or sweets or something third. Animals in the wild will do anything they can to lick the salt. From elephants to monkeys. If there is salt present anywhere in nature the animals will come to that place to lick it. It is called salt licking. In ancient times people and other predators used to wait for animals in these places so that they can hunt them. There are also artificial salt licks when people deliberately put salt to attract animals or maintain wildlife. We are the same and we as humans also lick salt, just in salted food. Refined salt is different than natural sea salt. Natural salt, unlike table salt, has trace minerals. Sea salt contains all of the trace minerals. In refined table salt, all of the trace minerals had been removed and now we will get just sodium and chloride and some added iodine. If you live in desert dry like conditions in high temperatures higher salt intake can have a beneficial role if you are sweating during the day because it will allow our body to store more water and will help against dehydration. In nature, it is very rare to find the salt unlike refined salt that we have today on every table but the instinct still remains in every animal.

A substance named ORMUS derived from a sea salt is the best and strongest organic natural fertilizer ever invented. It is considered as a natural organic fertilizer but it is expensive and commercially very hard to find. When I say ORMUS I don't mean monoatomic gold, David Radius Hudson type of ORMUS (Orbitally Rearranged Monoatomic Elements) but a natural fertilizer made out of regular unrefined sea salt that has all of the sea minerals in it. There is a type of historical, "mystical" ORMUS that is believed to be a form of monoatomic gold made by priest cast in Ancient Egypt and later it was experimented with in alchemical texts during Middle Ages and that is something completely different.

If you don't know what ORMUS historically is it might be a strange story for you. In ancient times it was believed to be an essence of eternal life. Alchemists through history were obsessing about creating gold. Most people don't realize that gold they are talking about is not real gold. In real Alchemy, they were trying to recreate what they call white gold. Nicolas Flamel for example in the last testament wrote about it and he is maybe the best-known alchemist from all time. This kind of monoatomic gold was not real gold because they were seeking the fountain of youth, not money. The objective of the alchemist had always been to make a "the container of the light of life" the "white powder of gold". If you partake of it, you live forever and so on. In Alchemy it all goes back to the man named Enoch. Also known as Hermes, Thoth, Trigeminus. Same man. He never died, instead ascended by partaking of the white drops because he was so perfect. If you ask a Rabbi about the white powder of gold, he will say that in Jewish tradition they have heard of it, but to their knowledge, no one has known how to make it since the destruction of the First Temple. The temple of Solomon. It was well known and recognized in history from Ancient Egypt to Assyria to Ancient Grease to Ancient Jewish tribes. Pharaohs would eat this gold and only Pharaohs not the rest of the people, and it was created by the special caste of the priesthood in the temples of workship (I didn't misspell this word). High Priest of Memphis held the title of Great Artificer. It was eaten as a wholly bread or when mixed with water it was known as "The Golden Tear from the Eye of Horus." You can see "Mfkzt" (sometimes pronounced "mufkuzt" the sacred bread or golden manna) in the Temple of Karnak for example. Now, this is recognized history not a fake. The word in Hebrew that means "What is it?" is translated literally into manna. When you play your next video game you will understand what manna really is. These stories are in the Bible in Exodus, in history, in alchemy, in ancient philosophy, and religion, and in ancient religious practices, and probably were practiced in Ancient Egypt in a real physical manner. In the ancient tradition of alchemy if you eat monoatomic powdered white gold you will experience superconductive abilities and for example you will have no need for energy anymore so you will be able to stop eating. The gifts that go with this are perfect telepathy, levitation, healing, resurrecting the dead within two or three days after they died and you would even have a strong aura that is visible and so on. That is why this is so interesting to people. If there is such a substance would you not want to have it? But in reality, monoatomic gold is just another scam. Or maybe not. I don't know. Nobody had done a real science and probably never would. It can be compelling for someone to start to use this kind of supplement.

In modern times it was rediscovered by Mr. Hudson who was a farmer and he began speaking publicly about his research and discoveries in 1995 and had one approved patent on his inventions but all of his claims were never scientifically verified to the full extent. He reportedly spent more than 8 million dollars in research. What Hudson believed is that his samples that he had collected from his land contained monoatomic gold because they will start to lose weight as cooled. This can only be possible if monoatomic gold or some other element in the sample have superconductive capabilities in the room temperature. Nevertheless, there are trace amounts of colloidal gold in the food. Actually, that is one way how you can find a gold line, if there are detectable particles of gold in any part of the tree. Big trees have big roots and if there is gold deep in the ground root of the tree will pick it up and if you test the organic matter from the tree you will see minute amounts of gold in colloidal form. Then you can prospect the land beneath. So yes we can eat colloidal gold but in nature, it would be in minuscule amounts so don't buy all of the secret alchemy fountain of youth new age stuff until real science is done. No one has monatomic gold as a commercial product today because the gold is very reactive. As soon as it cools it bounds itself with another molecule of gold. It can exist as a monoatomic particle but only in the Earth's core. When volcanoes in nature spill lava out there is monatomic gold in it. Maybe there is some way to produce monoatomic gold that is stable just by itself but I don't know. It is done by strong acid that will dissolve the pure refined gold to the monoatomic scale, then the acid is neutralized and then the monoatomic gold is refined from the solution. Me personally will not consume this supplement named ORMUS or ORME until science is done if its ever done. There were some experiments that were done in Lugano, Switzerland in the Alpha Learning Institute. The Alpha Learning Institute has the largest database in the world that correlates human performance with the degree of left-right brain balance and synchrony (over 35,000 EEG's). Simply stated, the more balanced the brain, the left and the right hemisphere connection, the easier it is to learn, there is higher IQ, more creativity, reduced anxiety, and improved mind-body coordination. Also, the more alpha waves are produced, the learning is easier and stress is lower. They gave a small amount of this substance to people in a clinical trial. The results were that it increased alpha wave pattern in the brain and there were increases in connectivity between brain hemispheres and the effects were cumulative. I will still take a break from this substance until further studies are done. If this is correct that it could be a treatment for ADD and ADHD and similar conditions. Most of us actually today in our regular life have higher left brain activity then the right one and I don't know why. What I do know is that many students these days will take Ritalin or Modafinil or just regular amphetamine to increase their mental capabilities.

But there is another type of ORMUS, Dead Sea salt ORMUS. Sodium and chloride are the most abundant ions in sea salt, representing about 33 and 50.9 percent of total minerals, respectively. Unlike refined table salt, sea salt is not 100 percent sodium and chloride. There is still depending on the source a range from less than 0.2 to 10 or more percent of other minerals in it. What you can do chemically is to remove sodium and chloride out of it and you will be left with just trace minerals and other minerals. Some people will drink this as a mineral supplement. Sea salt might also contain some heavy metals and microplastic and pollution but usually in a smaller amount than in sea animals due to bioaccumulation. What you can do is to put ORMUS on the ground as a fertilizer. This will give a big boost to the mineral composition of the soil. There are even some industrial operations that do this, extract minerals from sea salt as a fertilizer. And this will be considered organic fertilization by law. On the other hand, if you dump regular sea salt you will poison the land and nothing will grow on it for years. That is what Romans did to the Phoenician agricultural land during the Punic Wars to create famine and crop failure. You can use salt to kill plans in your back yard but that will be permanent and for years to come poisoning of the topsoil and after that nothing will grow. However, if you put ORMUS in the topsoil you will give a big boost to the plants and mineral composition of the soil. But this is expensive and most of the organic farmers will use just regular rock dust, manure, and wood ash. Rock dust is a very popular soil additive because it is cheap but it is not that effective because rock dust is just rock dust. Crushed stone.

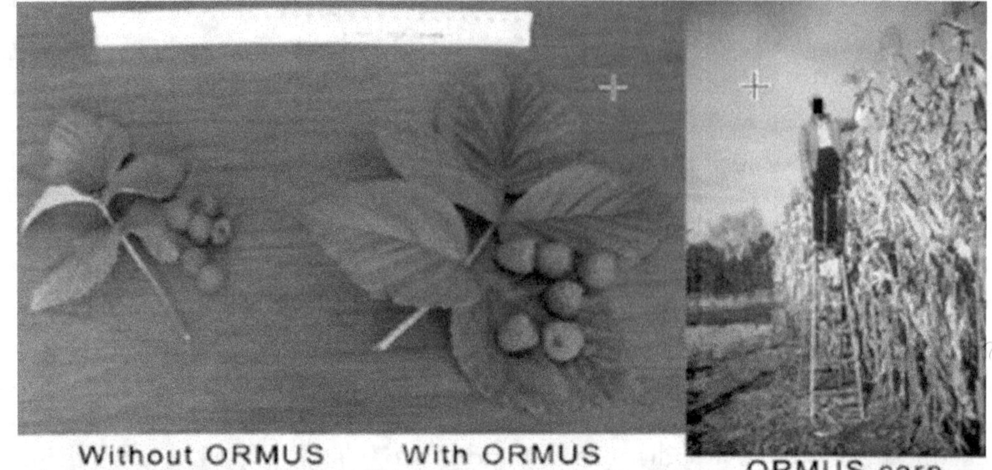

Without ORMUS   With ORMUS
ORMUS corn

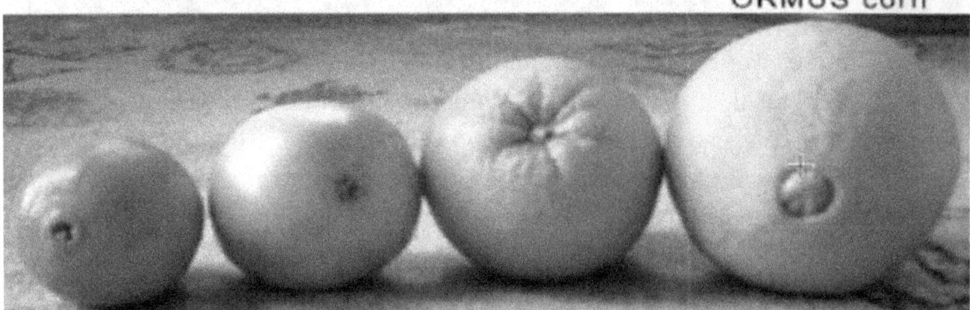

Ordinary orange   Ordinary grapefruit   2 year ORMUS orange   4 year ORMUS orange

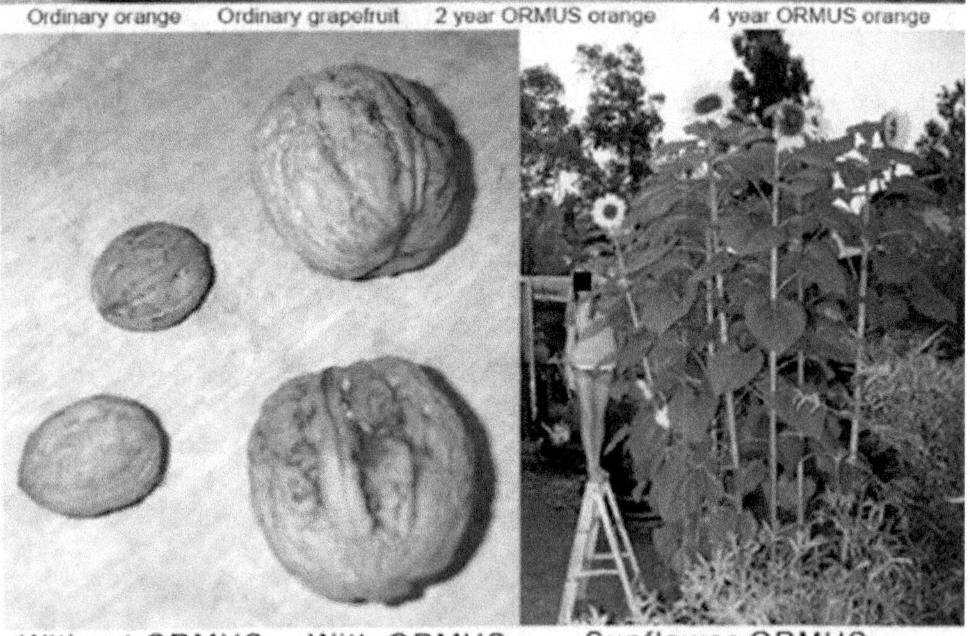

Without ORMUS   With ORMUS   Sunflower ORMUS

ORMUS is a colloidal mineral mixture, not a rock mixture. Big difference because ORMUS will be bioavailable for plant root systems to absorb it, but rock dust will not. Adding rock dust is similar to adding sand to the soil. It is possible that some of the minerals would leech from the rock dust to the soil but not in an adequate amount. The science does not support the use of rock dust and even the suppliers of rock dust suggest that it has no value in alkaline soil. Only in acidic soil the acid might dissolve some of the metals in it and make them bioavailable. But who will do this anyway? You will have to have your own garden and how many people have it? Food in stores is just completely nutrient deficient and filled with toxins and especially if you eat animal products you are in trouble. If you want to eat organic, you cannot. Food cannot be grown organically in large-scale production level for the entire population that exists in the world because most of the population want to eat animal products and most of the land is used for growing animal feed.

What we are left is just regular mineral deficient food and maybe some methods that we can use to increase the nutrient content of our diet. Trace minerals are the hardest to supplement. For example, boron helps the body to keep the calcium in the bone so that we do not get osteoporosis and helps the regulation of estrogen and can also raise testosterone in men. Who takes a boron supplement? Even if you do, supplements don't work. If you don't have enough boron you will have lower testosterone levels and I will assume that men know what that means and women will also suffer tremendously during the menopause. Chromium and vanadium are important for glucose metabolism. Without them, you will have insulin resistance or prediabetes symptoms and hypoglycemia. Who takes rare earth minerals as vanadium as a supplement? Most of the essential minerals such as magnesium, zinc and so on are deficient in most of the population nonetheless rare earth minerals.

The first symptoms of zinc deficiency are a loss of the sense of taste and smell. Zinc is a component of more than 2000 enzymes involved in digestion and metabolism including those for the breakdown of protein digestion, bone metabolism, alcohol, and phosphorus metabolism and the human genome encodes around 3000 zinc proteins (Zinc Biochemistry: From a Single Zinc Enzyme to a Key Element of Life doi:10.3945/an.112.003038). When you are zinc deficient, your body can't produce healthy, new cells. This leads to symptoms such as wounds that won't heal, open sores on the skin, lack of alertness and low energy, lowered immunity, infertility and growth retardation. In studies, the lowest intake of zinc was in young children aged 1-3 years (18.9%). 80 percent of young children in the U.S. were zinc deficient (Zinc Intake of the U.S. Population: Findings from the Third National Health and Nutrition Examination Survey, 1988-1994 doi.org/10.1093/jn/130.5.1367S). This study was conducted 20 years ago.

Around 12% of the adult population today is considered to be zinc deficient. To correct zinc deficiency high zinc fortification of breakfast cereals was implemented. Cereals is a food commonly eaten by children. Consequently, now 13 to 17 million American children are consuming amounts of zinc that exceed the tolerable upper intake levels set by the Institute of Medicine. And this is metallic inorganic zinc added as a supplement to the cereals for children. By now you should know what that means. 12 percent deficiency in adults is not bad and this is because there is a lot of zinc in some seafood, meat, and poultry.

However, a mineral that is mostly found in plant-based sources but is not present in animal products is magnesium. Chlorophyll in plants has the same molecular structure as hemoglobin with only one difference. Instead of magnesium in the center of a molecule of chlorophyll, there is iron so the color is red instead of green. As a consequence, the plant kingdom is going to have a lot more magnesium and the animal kingdom is going to have much more of the iron.

Hemoglobin

Chlorophyll

Thus if we have standard Western animal products dominated diet we will have a situation that around 61% of adults are magnesium deficient and 90 percent of teenagers. Nearly all known diseases are associated with a magnesium deficiency. It has so many functions in the body that the list is substantial. The mitochondria in cells heavily depend on magnesium to produce energy. Mitochondrial function mostly controls our energy levels. Because magnesium is involved in so many enzymatic processes in the body, a deficiency will obstruct over 300 normal processes. That is why it is hard to pinpoint magnesium deficiency. It can cause arrhythmias in the hart or fibromyalgia or migraine headache or muscle cramps or numbness and tingling or mood disorders. Magnesium deficiency also plays a key role in regulating neurotransmitter production. Magnesium is predominantly involved in GABA production in the brain, which is a calming neurotransmitter. A poor ability to produce adequate GABA levels results in conditions such as irritability, ADD/ADHD, anxiety, and depression. If you don't actively regulate your diet and control it and analyze it let me be the one to say this. You are having magnesium deficiency like most of the people. Because of the toxic overload in the body, the primary antioxidant that deals with all of the free radical and toxic damage and does a lot of detoxification is called glutathione. It is the primary antioxidant that our body creates. The problem is that you cannot make glutathione if you don't have magnesium (Effects of magnesium supplementation on the glutathione redox system in atopic asthmatic children. doi: 10.1007/s00011-007-7077-3). When you eat a lot of animal products you will consume a lot of toxins due to bioaccumulation, plus a lot of other toxins from the environment. At the same time, there will be a magnesium deficiency that will inhibit your body in natural detoxification mechanisms. Glutathione has a large number of biochemical reactions such as enzyme activation and DNA synthesis and repair. It can affect every cell in the body. Magnesium also affects adrenal glands and their hormonal response. When doctors correlate stress with some disease they forgot to mention that there is a step in between and that is magnesium deficiency both in terms of GABA production in the brain and in terms of hormonal effects and antioxidant capacity of the body. When your body is exposed to high levels of toxins and other stressors it will deplete magnesium quickly. Doctors will usually focus on the thyroid gland, calcium, and iron but somehow in the middle of all of this, they will forget adrenal glands and that magnesium deficiency affects 90 percent of young adults and teenagers and more than 60 percent of adults. For example, ATP (adenosine triphosphate), the main source of energy in cells, must bind to a magnesium ion in order to be biologically active. If you are taking creatine and are going to lift weights it would be a much better choice to balance your magnesium. Even osteoporosis or calcium deposits on the arteries or hyperparathyroidism that will cause high (primary hyperparathyroidism) or low (secondary hyperparathyroidism) calcium levels in the blood and other calcium issues might actually be magnesium deficiency. It is magnesium that regulates calcium metabolism. If you never heard about this ask yourself why? Today the countries with the highest calcium intake have the highest levels of osteoporosis. In Africa, women don't get osteoporosis on 300 mg of calcium per day but in Africa, they will eat a lot of calories from plant sources because they are poor and will have higher magnesium levels than average meat either. All three hormones that regulate calcium metabolism calcitonin (The relationship between magnesium and calciotropic hormones. Magnes Res. 1995 Mar;8(1):77-84.), parathyroid hormone (Magnesium modulates parathyroid hormone secretion and upregulates parathyroid receptor expression at moderately low calcium concentration doi: 10.1093/ndt/gft400) and active vitamin D metabolites, in particular, 1,25(OH)2 vitamin D3 (calcitriol) (Possible alterations of the in vivo 1,25(OH)2D3 synthesis and its tissue distribution in magnesium-deficient rats. Magnes Res. 1995 Mar;8(1):27-35.) are all regulated by magnesium. It might be strange to think that osteoporosis is actually magnesium deficiency, not calcium deficiency. Magnesium deficiency is associated with hypoparathyroidism, low production of active vitamin D metabolites, in particular, 1,25(OH)2 vitamin D3 and resistance to PTH and vitamin D. Even if you take vitamin D supplements they will not work without magnesium. This is exactly what we see in patients that have osteoporosis. Most of them will have high levels of calcium in the diet and will take supplemental vitamin D but will still be deficient in magnesium and will still develop osteoporosis and all of that excess calcium is going to give them calcium deposits instead of strong bones. It is hard to do a science of mineral balancing if you don't eat your normal plant foods and instead eat meat that has lower levels of magnesium. Even myself with a healthy diet had magnesium intake that was on the lower side but still manageable. I added cacao powder to my diet on a regular basis just because of the magnesium. And also cacao is full of antioxidants and other minerals as a bonus. If you eat grains and starch without too much of organic green leafy vegetables, you will have magnesium deficiency even if you are a vegan because of mineral-depleted soil. Meat, for example, has around 200 mg of magnesium for 1 kilogram of it and the RDA is 420 mg. It is impossible to eat enough magnesium on a meat-based diet. You would have to eat more than two kilograms of meat every single day and as a consequence would have a high and toxic intake of heme iron that is in excessive amounts a pro-radical and toxic substance to the body.

Non-heme iron, the iron found in plant foods is the iron usually regarded as less threatening because our bodies will decide if they need it and will lower or increase the absorption of it. Heme iron from meat is absorbed completely and can create toxicity in a prolonged period in meat dominated diets. Heme is a molecule that allows the iron to store oxygen in the body and it is a form of iron found in the animal kingdom only. RDA is 8 mg per day for males ages 19 and older and for example, clams have 23,8 mg per 3 oz. serving, Chicken Liver 8 mg for the same 3 ounces serving. To get to the recommended daily level of magnesium by eating 2 kg of beef meat you will ingest 42 mg of heme iron. If you have anemia taking an iron supplement is a waste of time and will just make your poop black. You will be just taking iron oxide or some other form of iron that is in inorganic form. Iron oxide is just rust and people are taking it as a supplement. It is an inorganic form of iron that is not absorbed well and even if it is absorbed it will just do damage because it is iron metal not iron in an organic bioavailable form. Also, a high iron intake will decrease copper and if you take an iron supplement you shut down copper metabolism. Adding C vitamin to an iron-rich meal will increase absorption (The role of vitamin C in iron absorption. Send to Int J Vitam Nutr Res Suppl. 1989;30:103-8). If you are worrying about iron deficiency on a plant-based diet, then just add some vitamin C rich fruit after the meal and that will take care of it. If you are vegan and pregnant then this can be an issue because a pregnant woman will have a higher demand for iron. Use this strategy and you will be fine. Why doctors push for awareness of calcium and iron and not magnesium is because they push milk for calcium and meat for iron and magnesium is in plants so it must be forgotten. Most people know about iron and calcium. It is true that calcium deficiency, for example, is correlated to more than 100 different diseases. But you can have as much calcium as you want if there are no hormones or enzymes in the body to put that calcium in the right spot it is of no use.

If I would to do a real full-blown analysis of every mineral for all of the science that is there, it would be a long book. It is almost impossible for you to know all of this. As an individual, you are only capable of governing your actions in a logical matter. You need to understand the principles that are in play here so that you can do rational thinking. If you want to science every molecule that would be impossible. There are rare earth minerals, that are known to have a biological functions that have been researched on laboratory animals. For example, have you ever heard about Thulium, Lanthanum, Neodymium, Praseodymium, Europium, Samarium, Ytterbium? All of those minerals are studied and we know that all of those minerals have some biological functions in our body. What exactly and how scientists don't know yet. The only conclusion that is made is that if you don't have them, and most of us don't, it would shorten the lifespan. Because we are so removed from nature we don't understand that the land where the crops are growing is not just some foreign object. It is in a direct sense the part of our body. Everything that is in that soil is going into you. The good, the bad and the ugly. Everything that is not in that soil and you need it is not going into you. You are, and I am, and we all are a part of nature no matter what some scientist is imagining. Average dog food will have around 40 minerals in it. The food they use as feed for laboratory rats will have 28 minerals in the rat pallets. They do regular laboratory testing of the nutrient content because bad nutrition is bad science. It could have a negative effect on studies if lab rats are deficient in some mineral. In some studies it can affect the result, so rat food for laboratory animals is of high quality. The highest quality you can get. How about our food. Average infant formula, and this had been tested, has 11 minerals in it in levels that are adequate. There will be listed on the label. Some came from milk some are added as a fortification. Cows are fed with corn that is grown on depleted soil and supplemented with some of the minerals that are needed but that is not natural and still, a big chunk of minerals will be missing. We have the situation that even laboratory rats have higher quality diets then human babies. Similac is called Similac because it lacks everything. It is a simulation. Simulating nature is a bad scientific practice. What about all of the other rare minerals that nobody tests or care about that are found in the fossil records of living organisms? We won't die immediately from deficiency but they do something in our body so we might just have chronic diseases and shorten lifespan even if we do get iron and calcium and magnesium.

Plants have the ability to make most of the vitamins and amino acids and essential fats. They will take carbon out of the air and make all of these molecules using solar energy. You will have to eat different whole plant foods to take different nutrients and it is possible. The problem is most of the developed world has a low-quality diet and most of the calories are coming from refined foods with no nutritional value. On top of that even bigger problem is that plants cannot transform the solar energy into the solid matter like minerals. Minerals have to be present in the ground to be broken down into organic form and used. Longevity is achieved by evolutionary congruent lifestyle with a healthy diet and physical activity. People in the rural parts of the world have the longest and the healthiest lives without Medicare or hospitals. When you look for example at Hunza people most of them don't even have sanitation and still live to 100 with no heart disease, cancer, stroke, diabetes or obesity. Imagine that. When you put NPK on the land, meaning nitrogen, phosphorus, and potassium you will get those three minerals in the finished produce. It takes only 5 to 10 years to deplete minerals from the soil with this practice. Only 10 years. The ones of the most prosperous people in antiquity were Egyptians. They glorified the river Nile as a divinity because it would cause a flood every year. With flood also comes the mud full and rich with different kinds of minerals so they didn't have to put any form of fertilizer to the soil and would always have a successful harvest with constant and high yields of crops. That is the reason why the entire Egyptian civilization was basically living in the Nile River delta and didn't spread anywhere else. In other places in the world people would be burning forests and then in that ash they would plant the crops. When that topsoil was depleted then they would just burn some more of the forest and because the number of people was extremely low that would work. Plus, some foraging and hunting and fishing and that was it. Today we use 40 percent of the entire habitable planet landmass for ourselves. I don't count deserts, Siberia, Antarctic, and Greenland. But from all of the landmass that can be cultivated 40 percent is already in use by people in terms of construction and other infrastructure and for agriculture and other forms of industries. Monoculture and artificial fertilization with NPK is the only feasible option.

Usually, everyday people will have an idea to take a lot of supplements as a correction. It is always the case but let us do some real analysis. Let's do calcium analysis for example. We need 1000mg per day. The industry has no way to create organic or colloidal calcium, or let say it in this way, the industry has no economically feasible way of producing bioavailable calcium so they will just sell some metallic form of it or chelated metallic form of it and that is just a scam. But let's do some math. If you take for example 1000mg of calcium lactate (usually 2 tablets). Only 250mg of that 1000mg calcium lactate is calcium in metallic form. The rest of it is lactate. And then because it is a metallic form of calcium stomach acid might dissolve some of it so average absorption will be around 10%. That 10% is also problematic because absorbed calcium molecule might be still too big to do any biochemical action in the body but let say all 10 percent are ionized by the stomach acid and bioavailable. You will end up with 25mg of calcium in the bloodstream from 1000mg of calcium tablet. If you take the chelated form of calcium to get better absorption you will just end up with a large amount of metallic calcium in your blood and that is just by itself toxic. There are some minerals that are bioavailable in supplemental form but calcium is not one of them. If you want a supplement to do the job of the food you will have to take 80 of those 500mg calcium lactate tablets. And after that, you still have 64 minerals to go.

The reason why for example the Hunza people or people that are long-lived don't have mineral deficiencies that live in high altitudes is speculated to be due to the glacial water. This water in Tibet is called glacial milk. There is no rain in that altitudes except for glacial water. In Tibet, they have less than two inches of precipitation in a year. Glaciers will grind up rocks and will have rock dust infused with water and some of the minerals would be in colloidal form. Glaciers usually exert huge amounts of pressure on the rocks and water will pick up this grinded metallic rock dust. People will use that water to irrigate the fields. They will also drink it. Plants will pick up some of the minerals from that water and will make them into a bioavailable organic form. In the time period of thousands of years, the soil will be constantly infused with glacial milk water and will remain in good condition and will not have mineral depletion. At least this is just a theory. The real scientific test was never done or I didn't find any. In Europe and in other colder climates the practice before electricity was always the same. People will be burning wood for heating of the houses and they will be using that ash that is just minerals from the wood as a fertilizer. The usual practice was to dump the ash into the garden. The ash will infuse the soil with minerals and the soil would have good yields every year.

Today nobody knows or talks about the importance of minerals. In medicine, they have a belief that genetic is the most important deciding factor, not some mineral deficiency. Then the next most important issue would be nerve transmitters and neuroscience in general. Then endocrine system with all of the hormones in the body. Then the immune system. Then at the end of the line, they will talk about enzymes and then vitamins. Minerals are forgotten and I will say on purpose. You can have a gene therapy or hormonal therapy or some patented enzymes therapy but how are you going to make a profit from something that cannot be patented? There is a reason why minerals are considered to be of less importance than all other areas in medicine and that is not by accident. In the current state that we are in, the situation is exactly inverted. Mineral deficiency is the root cause of many diseases alongside unnatural evolutionary maladapted lifestyle and diet. Nobody will advise people to lower animal products consumption and to take care of mineral deficiencies. They will say to people it is all just some bad genes or something else here take some drugs. Medical doctors themselves or let say many of them have no idea of the importance of mineral balancing. They are not trained in medical school to treat the root causes of diseases but only just symptoms with different drugs and surgery. Vitamins will not work without minerals. Minerals must be present in order for vitamins to work. And when they are present in medicine they are called coenzymes. Many people don't understand what enzymes in the body actually are. They are vitamins plus amino acids plus minerals that have a chemical reaction to make enzymes and then enzymes have influence and create some process in the body. If one of three is missing the entire process doesn't work. Hormones in the body and neurotransmitters in the brain are made out of enzymes. If we are deficient in zinc or magnesium or copper the genes cannot work properly. It is the minerals that run the show.

Mineral competition wheel

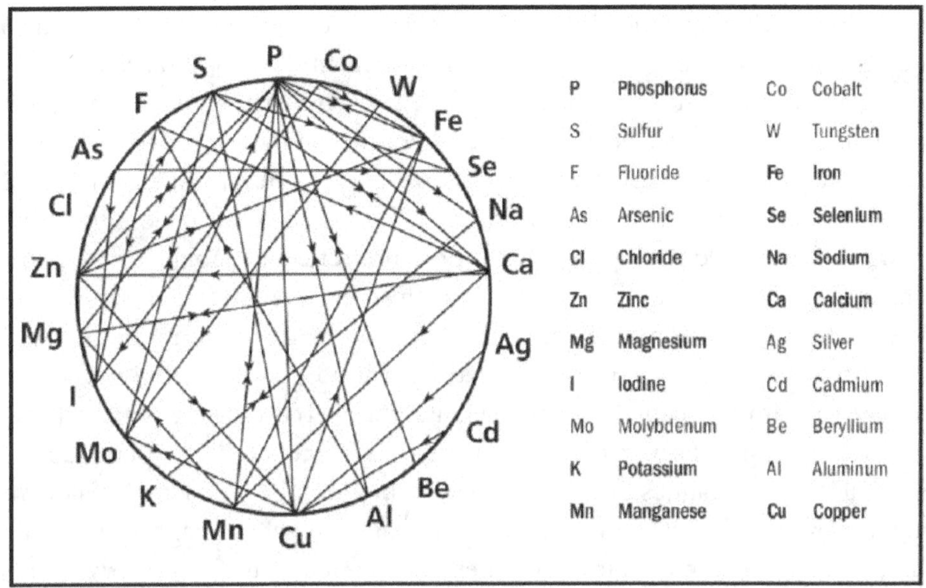

Every mineral has opposing mineral and that is a big issue. The excess amount of one can cause dysfunction of another mineral. Usually, people know about for example zinc and copper, or sodium and potassium or already mention magnesium and calcium. Why excess sodium will give you bloat is not because of the sodium but because of the lacking of potassium. So it is actually the balance of the sodium and potassium that is disrupted with excess sodium. It is in fact unopposed sodium, not sodium that is creating water retention in the body. Paleolithic hunter-gatherers consumed about 11,000 milligrams of potassium a day from vegetables, roots, leaves, fruits and other plant sources, and well under 700 mg of sodium. That's a sodium-to-potassium ratio of 1 to 16. Today, we have table salt everywhere for an average of 3,400 mg of sodium in a day and in some cases much more than that and around 2,500 mg of potassium, for a ratio of 1.36 to 1. In comparison, our ancestors lived by foraging and sweating in a climate of Africa.

Creating perfect balance in the body is hard especially if you eat a diet that is not in line with our evolution with industrially grown crops on mineral-depleted soil. The best thing you can do is to analyze your diet for a month. There are fitness programs that have charts for calorie needs and for most of the RDA nutrients and then after a month, you will have an insight into the mineral composition of your diet. Then you can make the correction by adding food items that are rich in the nutrient that you are lacking. The best course of action is to cut most of the animal products and add high-quality whole plant foods instead. And then analyze again and correct again. If you don't want to do all of this, you can give your hair for mineral analysis. A serum blood test is not accurate because our body needs to have a constant pH of the blood of 7.35 to 7.45 and uses minerals for balancing. Minerals can show to be in relatively normal levels in the blood but hair test will give you a real tissue measure of mineral levels. If you have all of the minerals in normal ranges and don't have deficiencies, then you can look at the different ratios to see if everything is in balance. A nutritional expert can have a look at specific ratios of minerals. For example, the calcium/potassium ratio of less than 4:1 is indicative of increased thyroid activity. It does not reflect the ability of the thyroid to make T4 or T3 hormones (as a blood test does). Instead, it reflects how efficiently the T3 hormone can access each cell. When this action is inhibited, the result is fatigue. This would be indicated by a ratio greater than 18 where the excessive calcium is creating reduced cellular permeability. A low ratio reflects a sensitivity to sugar indicative of excessive thyroid effect and highly permeable cell walls. Calcium to magnesium ratio is also a blood sugar indicator. Calcium is required for the release of insulin from the pancreas while magnesium inhibits insulin secretion. A high ratio indicates the tendency to improperly manage calcium and this can lead to deposits in abnormal places in the body. A low ratio usually indicates a calcium deficiency. As calcium is required and utilized by the pancreas to make insulin, a high or low ca/mg ratio (over 10:1 or under 3:1) indicates a tendency towards diabetes and a diet high in refined sugars and carbohydrates. But then again cortisone therapy will lower calcium levels and lead and cadmium toxicity will displace calcium. These types of tests are not something you can read by yourself, you will have to go to the clinic that specializes in this type of analysis. There are seven of these types of ratios that can be indicative of disease trends. These ratios are not diagnostic but are research associations. But if you are below RDA for some of the minerals then the first thing you need to do is to correct that deficiency by adding the foods that are rich in that particular mineral. Produce also has to be organically grown without artificial fertilizers. The problem is that there are 65 minerals and most of them do not have RDA. Science does not even know what some of these minerals even do in the body. However, when you go to the regular doctor's office because of let say anemia or osteoporosis the standard treatment will be to supplement with iron or calcium. That approach can have a negative effect on the body because the approach is not holistic and the MDs are not trained to heal people holistically. Taking iron will not heal your anemia and taking calcium will not heal osteoporosis. The opposite mineral of calcium is magnesium. So, when you have toxicity or deficiency of one mineral you also have disrupted the level of opposite mineral. Too much calcium will create magnesium deficiency and magnesium is needed to create enzymes that are responsible for calcium metabolism in the first place. Magnesium deficiency will create osteoporosis just by itself and we already discussed why.

Too much copper will create zinc deficiency for example. The opposite mineral of copper is zinc. When you have too much copper your MD is going to do his best to detox all of that excess copper because excess copper is toxic especially to the brain and many other organs. In our body, there are about 30 enzymes that are dependent on copper metabolism. Our body cannot make connective tissue and bones without copper or neurotransmitters or part of the immune system or cellular energy in the form of ATP. ATP (Adenosine triphosphate) creation depends on copper metabolism and taking creatine as a supplement won't do you much good if you are copper deficient. If you have high copper levels dosing with zinc might not be a good idea if you are not zinc deficient. High levels of copper can be a result of three different deficiencies, not just zinc. Copper exists and this is unique for copper and in some way for iron too, in bout active and bound form. Ceruloplasmin is the enzyme that bounds to copper in the blood, and in addition, play a role in iron metabolism. It turns the copper into a bioavailable form, to a different state with a different electrical charge. So copper toxicity can be caused by ceruloplasmin levels. Too much of it and you have too much copper, too little of it and you have low levels of copper. If you have high copper levels it can also be an unusable form of copper that does nothing except creating problems. For example, you have consumed a lot of copper-containing foods but have low levels of ceruloplasmin you could end up with high levels of unusable copper in the bloodstream and low levels of copper in the cells. If you have low usable copper it also means you have low usable iron and then you are anemic. So, taking an iron supplement means nothing. Copper toxicity hides three different states of deficiencies. When testing for copper you should always test for both forms in the blood. High levels of copper in the blood can actually be low levels of iron, low levels of zinc and low levels of usable bioavailable copper. If you are anemic and the doctor tells you to take an iron supplement and he didn't test for copper, he is not familiar with this science and will do you a lot of harm. Your ferritin might go up but that is it. You will still be anemic. For anemia, for example, you might have to eat whole food bioavailable copper that is known as vitamin C. Whole food vitamin C has a copper in it. When you read about the increase in non-heme iron absorption caused by vitamin C it is also an increase of bioavailability of iron in general not just about absorption if you have dysregulation in copper metabolism. An enzyme that turns plant iron into heme animal form of iron also depends on copper. Protoporphyrin IX is the enzyme that creates the heme when complexed with ferrous iron so that heme iron is able to store oxygen. To make a ferrous iron body needs a Ferroxidase enzyme. If copper is not bioavailable the body will not be able to make ferroxidase enzyme to make the heme, to make the heme iron, to make the hemoglobin. If you have high or low copper the key is to increase the bioavailability of copper not just to take some drug that will detoxify your blood out of excess copper. Doing that is not going to help you in the long run if you don't increase the bioavailability of copper. If you have iron or copper issues you should test for ceruloplasmin levels. There is no iron metabolism without copper. It is copper iron metabolism. Iron is not designed to be deposited anywhere inside the body. Around 80 percent of the iron is found in hemoglobin and not in free form. Less than 10 percent is found in ferritin inside the cells and not running through the blood. The study by Vanoaica, et al (2010) found that Ferritin-H is needed for accurate control of iron levels. Ferritin-H has ferroxidase enzyme function, so copper is needed at the end to regulate iron levels in the same way that magnesium is needed to regulate calcium metabolism.

People who are under stress can lose a lot of magnesium and are deficient in the first place because of high animal product low green leafy vegetables rich in chlorophyll diet. And then when they lose the magnesium the anterior pituitary gland will start to pump ACTH (Adrenocorticotropic hormone) that is produced in a response to biological stress. ACTH causes the liver to stop making the ceruloplasmin. Also, when you take a lot of calcium not just zinc it will block copper absorption in the gut. And then the ceruloplasmin that regulates copper requires the copper itself to be made in the first place. Ceruloplasmin contains six atoms of copper in its structure. If you take too much vitamin D, you can drop the bioavailable copper levels as well. When you take vitamin D you are also wiping out vitamin A in the liver and it takes vitamin A in order to make ceruloplasmin. You see now how bad all of this can be. When we start to live and eat in a way that is not congruent with our evolution taking iron for anemia or calcium for osteoporosis or taking medication for copper toxicity that you will get in the prescription from any licensed MD is just making things even worse. For example, when you take ascorbic acid is not natural vitamin C. It is the main part of it but there are other molecules in there like copper. Taking ascorbic acid will actually make copper less bioavailable but taking natural vitamin C will make copper more bioavailable and natural vitamin C has the copper in it in the first place. In natural vitamin C, there is an enzyme called tyrosinase and this enzyme will enable the body to use copper ions from vitamin C. The enzyme is also involved in melanin synthesis so it can create albinism or hyperpigmentation. Using ascorbic acid as an inhibitor of tyrosinase activity has been utilized in cosmetics for the conditions related to the hyperpigmentation of the skin, such as melasma and age spots but eating it in excessive amounts can create a copper deficiency. Even something like vitamin C can have different effects on the body depending on the molecular form of which that vitamin is in.

The question that we should ask is are we able to science every molecule to the end and know all of the science in our everyday life? Reading books on nutrition can help you but not in a way most people would like. Taking pills for everything cannot work and allopathic form of medicine cannot work. Sooner or later allopathic medicine and sciencing of every enzyme, every gene, everything that exists in the body would lead to a holistic approach such as mineral balancing, diet balancing and so on. Just taking pills or extracted chemicals can never work to the full extent and in most cases is bad to the health. For example, high fructose corn syrup in the extracted form will cause a drop in liver copper and increase in liver iron levels which will then prevent the production of ceruloplasmin. Excess heme iron from meat and iron supplements will also cause the suppression of ceruloplasmin production as well. Because we have too much meat in the diet, we will have too much heme iron in the diet and that will then prevent the production of ceruloplasmin. If there is an excess amount of unusable copper it will build up in the tissues and will create tissue damage. For example, copper accumulation in the brain will cause a tremor of the hands and extremities that is permanent and cannot be cured. At the same time, bioavailable copper would not be in the cells and will not be there to create neurotransmitters. Then low dopamine levels in the brain (the feel-good chemical), will give you addictive behavior cravings and personality disorder. It will make you crave alcohol and other forms of drugs and foods that stimulate dopamine receptors in the brain. It will force you to eat excessively and compulsively and will create other forms of compulsive behaviors just so that you can feel good or normal. One of the main reasons might be dopamine deficiency. The brain creates dopamine with amino acid tyrosine and enzyme dopamine beta-monooxygenase (DBH). DBH contains copper. DBH has been implicated as a correlating factor in conditions associated with decision making, alcoholism, addictive drugs and smoking, schizophrenia, attention deficit hyperactivity disorder, and Alzheimer's disease. Copper plus tyrosine makes dopamine. No bioavailable copper, no dopamine. If you have an alcoholic in the family, you might want to test for mineral deficiencies. And when you start to drink alcohol it will burn out substantial amounts of magnesium and zinc and B vitamins in the body. And then when this happens it will suppress the production of ceruloplasmin. Then that will lower the bioavailability of copper and then that will create dopamine deficiency and then that will create alcohol, sugar and other cravings for addictive substances. It is a nice self-sustaining loop. If you suffer from let's say magnesium deficiency you are going to be agitated and filled with anxiety and have stressful life with problems and feelings of hopelessness. People don't want to believe that their mental state can be altered just by diet regime. Most of the people want some sort of reinforcement that they are self-controlling and above "stupid" things like diet. Especially when doctors stick labels like you have manic depression or you are alcoholic or you are suffering from gamble addiction. Here are some nice magic pills for you that will make you even more depressed in the long run. And the truth is completely inverted. You are magnesium deficient and have high levels of iron from meat and that affects your brain chemistry and all other minerals are deficient too and no drugs or surgery will help you. It is not normal for any other animal in nature including primates to suffer from these types of behaviors but today we are exposed to supernormal stimuli in form of food every single day and are eating meat instead of magnesium-rich green leafy vegetables filled with chlorophyll. In the end, this is all because of mineral-depleted soil and excessive animals products consumption. If you don't want to believe this do your own research. Mineral deficiencies will create a never-ending cascade of bad effects. And we are just talking here about eating meat and junk.

What happens when we add all of the toxic metals from the polluted environment to the picture like mercury, cadmium, and aluminum. I already analyzed this in the first part of the series so I will not go into details here. One thing that I did not explain is that these heavy metals, especially mercury and aluminum, disrupt antioxidant metabolism in the liver. There are three enzymes that our body uses as antioxidant protection against free radical damage that are created internally. These are superoxide dismutase, catalase, and glutathione peroxidase. Copper and zinc are essential for superoxide dismutase created inside the cells (SOD 1) and manganese is essential for superoxide dismutase created in mitochondria (SOD2). Catalase depends on iron. It contains four iron-containing heme groups but again iron is only good as copper is as good. Glutathione peroxidase in all mammalian forms are selenium-containing enzymes but also requires magnesium to be created. Also, it does not work as well in a copper-deficient organism and they don't know why. But wait how many of us have selenium or magnesium deficiency. Basically entire European continent is selenium deficient and 90 percent of young adults and teenagers are magnesium deficient. What this means is low levels of glutathione peroxidase and high levels of oxidative damage and inflammation especially with all of the toxic overload we are exposed to. This will lead to chronic inflammation and all of the diseases that come along with it like cancer for example. Most of the diseases we have today are caused by the single thing and that is not something that dropped from outer space. It is a shift in diet. That is it. We are designed by 60 million years of evolution to eat vegan whole food diet. Medical students will not learn this in college. The ones that do are the specialists that have a job in laboratories and not with patients so there is ignorance on both sides of the stethoscope.

I will recap some basic biochemistry in the most unscientific way that I can to simplify all of this. Nature is a closed system where balance exists. Any action that is not in the line of evolutionary biology or in other words our own nature will create health problems. In nature plants use photosynthesis and this is just the process of splitting water (H_2O) into Hydrogen and Oxygen to create energy

(ATP). This allows the plants to live. Animals do the exact opposite. Humans and other animals combine hydrogen and oxygen to make water (H2O) in order to create energy (ATP). This process requires bioavailable copper and also ensures that excess iron leaves the body. If we have too much iron, we would have inflammation and cellular damage. Excess iron can make havoc inside us. Copper makes H2O and releases ADP (not ATP), which is a precursor of ATP. Then ADP joins up with magnesium to create Mg-ATP, the active chemical of energy that the cells recognize and use. Because we have shifted from magnesium-rich plant foods to heme iron-rich animal flesh we have 60 to 90 percent magnesium deficient population. This creates problems because our body needs to be able to create energy and clear the exhaust. Magnesium or the bioavailable copper depleted body can't make enough energy. This will create inflammation that is chronic and will result in cascading of negative effects already mentioned. I always ask people who want my advice what is real food? Most of them had no idea what real food is. Most of the younger generations had no idea what food is nonetheless real food. So what is real food? The answer is the food that does not have any label on top of it. The food that you can eat without any preparation. The food that does not have any chemical added to it or to the soil. The food you will find by foraging. That is real food. Not a mineral depleted chemical list filled with toxins.

How can we get enough magnesium? We can look at RDA but that is just an estimate by the government agency that might be intentionally low. For example, to avoid any manipulation of the data we can look at fossil records. All of those paleo, keto diet people when confronted with facts like this have no real answer. In the Paleolithic nutrition of the former hunter/gatherers, they had a magnesium uptake with the usual diet of about 600 mg of magnesium/day. Hunting wild beast and eating cooked flesh was a new invention for them that Homo erectus didn't do so even them that had started to eat flesh still get around 600mg of magnesium. Hominids before them have eaten much more. If you want to do a real paleo diet go ahead and design a diet that will have at least 600 mg of magnesium a day and I will have no problem with that. Magnesium comes in a package. When you eat a whole food without using supplements to get to the 600 mg of it you will have to take a lot of calories and you will find soon enough that it is impossible to eat meat and animal products more than 5 to 10 percent of calories to get to this number. That is a real paleo diet that was just by itself unnatural and a new invention. In the time period of 30 to 50 million years before that hominins haven't consumed flesh at all. Today in developed countries with the Western diet, the average intake of magnesium is slightly over 4 mg/kg/day. That is about 300 mg for adult and that is just by looking at charts and not taking into account that most of the soil is depleted and that these charts don't represent the real values if the food is not grown organically in mineral-rich soil. You cannot take 600mg of magnesium in a day if you eat any amount of animal products, period. To take 600 mg of magnesium you will have to rely on whole foods organically grown plant-based diet. One kg of lean beef meat has 170mg of magnesium on average. Let me write this again. One kg of lean beef red meat has 170 mg of magnesium. But it would also have 26 mg of heme iron, and that is toxic, extremely toxic and pro-inflammatory to the body. One liter of milk will have around 100mg of magnesium. All of the misguided keto paleo diet people who want to argue with me and with themselves have a simple task. Go ahead and eat all animal products and whatever you like as long as you take 600 mg of magnesium without any supplements and do not surpass RDA for iron. All you need is 300 grams of beef to surpass RDA for iron and then you would not be allowed to eat anything else. Western diet may provide enough magnesium to avoid frank magnesium deficiency, but it is unlikely to maintain high-normal magnesium levels and provide optimal risk reduction from coronary artery disease and osteoporosis and other magnesium deficiency diseases. Here is one quote (Vormann J. Magnesium: nutrition and metabolism. Mol Aspects Med 2003;24:27-37.doi:10.1016/S0098-2997(02)00089-4): "At least 300 mg magnesium must be supplemented to establish significantly increased serum magnesium concentrations." " Only American diets containing more than 3000 kcal/day may provide 300 mg or more magnesium." (Lakshmanan FL, Rao RB, Kim WW, et al. Magnesium intakes, balances, and blood levels of adults consuming self-selected diets. Am J Clin Nutr 1984;40:1380-9). It is not me saying this it is a well-accepted scientific fact and it is easy to check for yourself. RDA for magnesium (between 300 and 420 mg/day for most people) is just designed to prevent frank magnesium deficiency. Why is there all of the stories about calcium and iron and so on when most of the population already consumes high and in some cases the toxic amounts of calcium and iron that will create calcium deposits in the body and heme iron toxicity? Lakshmanan et al found that the mean magnesium intake was 323 mg/day and 234 mg/day in men and women, respectively (around 4 mg/kg/day). Moreover, 75% of women consumed less than the RDA (300 mg/day). Intake of magnesium in Germany, for example, was determined to be only 200 mg for women and 250 mg for men. If we start to eat a lot of meat and other animal products and start to eat a lot of empty calories like sugar or oil and then have mineral-depleted soil what is a consequence? Nutrient deficiency and chronic disease.

The importance of the mineral content of the soil was once understood by farmers but with technology and a shift in our diet after the Industrial Revolution, we have a big problem. Only when the consequence is physically visible the industry will do something. If the problem is silent and chronic then there will be no interest in public awareness. Remember the story of low iodine levels in soil and the increased prevalence of goiter. It is a story mostly forgotten today and people believe they have adequate iodine intake if they don't have a visible goiter. There are two different types of goiter. The thyroid hypertrophy where the TSH stimulates thyroid cells and then there is goiter that is caused by iodine deficiency where there is hyperplasia (increase in the amount of tissue that results from cell division). Because of hyperplasia individuals that have goiter also have a higher rate of some types of cancer like breast cancer and ovaries and thyroid cancer. In past times due to the fact that iodine is easily washed away from topsoil and eventually ends up in oceans, there was a worldwide deficiency that caused the pregnant woman to have children with mental retardation. Cretinism or correct name today would be congenital iodine-deficiency syndrome is caused by iodine deficiency during fetus development that is causing thyroid hormone deficiency and then indirectly mental retardation. Now if you have slight iodine deficiency your baby might not have total retardation but just lowered IQ. This was a big problem and for example in the Great Lakes region in the 1900s more than 40 percent of children had a goiter. Because of this, there was a law passed that forced mandatory iodine supplementation by adding it to the table salt. Usually, the ratio of women to a man that has hypothyroidism is 9 to 1. More women will have goiter then men and the reason is estrogen. Estrogen inhibits the absorption of iodine. Also in iodine deficiency, ovarian estrogen production increases and estrogen receptor number in breast tissue also increases which then creates the risk of breast cancer especially if you drink milk or eat dairy products that are filled with estradiol and other androgenic hormones. But the real mystery here is, how is it possible that the human organism has as such high necessity to iodine if the iodine is not present at that level in the soil? Some of the theories for this that anthropologists have is that our hominins ancestors started to live in the big deltas near the coast of oceans as an intermediate niche after the forests were gone in Africa due to climate change. Because of the barren savanna land, they might have started to eat a lot more of sea vegetables that were found on the ocean coast. This is just a thesis however the amount of iodine that we currently need is much more then we can possibly get by our regular diet if we don't eat sea vegetables on a daily basis.

It is not just a thyroid gland that uses iodine to make hormones. Every cell in our body needs iodine. White blood cells, for example, need iodine to function properly. They use iodine to fight infections. Iodine deficiency is linked to cancer. Iodine is found in the skin, brain, breast, pancreas, ovaries and so on. Thyroid has a large deposit for iodine but outside of thyroid gland ovaries also have the ability to make thyroid hormone. T3 just means that there are 3 atoms of iodine that are bound together and T2 means that there are 2 atoms of iodine bound together. If you have thyroid issues doctor will also test the ovaries. Ovaries do not make T3 just T2. But T2 can be used by the body to make T3 or T4. The only difference is that ovaries cannot store the iodine as thyroid can. It is common to see women gaining weight when their ovaries start to fail because of the decrease in T2 production. Another tissue that concentrates iodine is salivary glands. If you don't have enough iodine you cannot make saliva. Your throat and eyes will go dry and that will create an infection. Breast concentrates a lot of iodine and iodine there has an antiseptic role in milk secretion for the baby. Lack of iodine in the breast will cause an increased risk of breast cancer. Almost 20 percent of all iodine stored in the body goes to the skin. Lack of iodine in the skin will cause dryness. Also, you would not be able to sweat and would be prone to sensitivity and infections especially if you have some cut or wound. Iodine is antiseptic and that is why it is used by all the glands that need to create something that is sterile like a mother's milk or embryo or to protect the skin. In surgeries, for example, iodine is also used as a disinfection agent and for wounds and injuries as well. Iodine in the brain will make us more mentally alert. If you take an iodine supplement before you go to bed you will have trouble going to sleep.

How much iodine do we actually need? There is no answer. The reality is that we do not know how much exactly but we can make the correct approximation. The current RDA for iodine is 150 mcg for adult female and 220 mcg for a pregnant female. That is micrograms. One milligram has 1000 mcg. This is the number given by the FDA and this is the number that is so low that it is almost absurd what this governmental agency is pushing for. Why they are doing this I don't know but I can speculate. This is a number that is the lowest number that will allow our body to avoid goiter and visible mental retardation. The lowest possible number that is far away from optimal and real physiological necessity. MD's will disagree with me but we will understand why and how much we really need if we look at some real numbers. It is true that taking iodine in specific illnesses like hypothyroidism and autoimmune thyroid disease will allow the thyroid gland that is not working properly to disrupt the levels of hormones in the bloodstream. That is not the iodine fault but the malfunction of the gland itself. If you have a normal thyroid gland there will be no hypothyroidism because the gland is functioning properly and you will not have to worry about it. You can take as much iodine as you want it would not create hypothyroidism. It would just be excreted out of the body. The real truth is that if a person suddenly consumes an enormous amount of iodine nothing will happen. Normally functioning thyroid gland will "shut off" its import of iodine and that is it. It will stop producing thyroid hormone temporarily. This is called the "Wolff-Chaikoff Effect". This will be a normal response from normal functioning thyroid to stop the overproduction of hormones so that the gland can upregulate or downregulate the receptors, enzymes, and other processes involved with iodine. It's considered a normal homeostasis response. The thyroid gland is doing this all the time, every day and it is completely normal. You cannot shut down a thyroid completely with dietary iodine intake even if you want to. This process happens with other cells as well. If higher iodine intake continues for an extended period of time the body will adapt to it with no problems with no consequence if you have normal functioning of other enzymes and thyroid gland. Iodine will be excreted by the kidneys instead of being captured by the thyroid gland but only after you have saturated your entire body. If an individual is getting too little iodine the opposite will happen, iodine will be recycled in the body instead of being excreted by the kidneys. The thyroid that is completely deficient might even do the initial overstimulation of thyroid hormone production in extremely rare cases if there is no autoimmune disease. If a person has been iodine deficient their entire life and suddenly there is an increase in iodine consumption, the thyroid gland will "turn on" full throttle to try to capture this iodine. There is a reserve of iodine in the thyroid and in initial stages until this reserve is filled the thyroid will keep taking as much iodine as it can until homeostatic regulation kicks in and normal function of the thyroid is achieved. So, in some individuals, sudden iodine supplementation might cause sudden and initial hypothyroidism because of high TSH that will be subclinical. In the "old days", both potassium iodide and Lugol's Iodine were used to treat Grave's disease, which is hyperthyroidism (overproduction). A normal reaction to the iodine supplementation can be to shut down the thyroid and cause hypothyroidism temporarily. For example, patients undergoing thyroidectomies may be given potassium iodide in large amounts right before surgery and for 10 days before the surgery as well. Large amounts (milligrams) of potassium iodide will "shut down" the thyroid gland temporarily. Temporarily being the keyword. Only when a person develops thyroid problems, like autoimmune thyroid diseases such as thyroiditis, Hashimoto, and Grave's disease, as well as thyroid cancer or autonomously functioning nodules, all bets are off. The normal homeostatic mechanisms that should keep the body in balance no longer work very well, or at all.

The thyroid gland just by itself has the ability to store 50 mg of iodine. That is milligrams not micrograms. It is 50,000 mcg and RDA is 150 mcg. Does this seem normal to you? How about this. Our entire body has the ability to store 1,500 mg of iodine. That is 1,500,000 mcg of iodine and the RDA is 150 mcg. Does this seem normal to you? You can take as much iodine as you want until this body reserve is not filled you will not have excess iodine problem. Can we fill our iodine body reserve of 1,500,000 mcg of iodine with 150 mcg a day? For instance, 32 percent of our body's iodine stores are in our muscles. Unlike other metallic minerals, iodine can be dissolved in plain water so there is no need for enzymatic detoxification. It can be excreted easily by the urine. That is exactly the reason why iodine is so easily washed away from the topsoil and why it will end up in ocean water. It can also take a monoatomic form like water and evaporate to form a gas. That is the smell of the ocean. It is just the evaporated iodine. Once airborne, iodine combines with evaporated water particles in the air and drops back to the soil near the coast and back to the ocean and will never reach far back to the main continent where it has been initially. It remains in the ocean water permanently. Our hominin ancestors that lived near the ocean coast consumed much more iodine in the diet than us. The good news is that it is one of the rare minerals that can be completely bioavailable if taken in the supplemental form. There are actually two types of iodine that our body uses iodine and iodide but you don't have to know all of this. Dietary iodine, such as the one found in seaweed, is present in the iodide form (bound to potassium to form a salt), as is the iodine in iodized salt. Taking just potassium iodide is enough because there is an enzyme in the specific organs to convert one form into another depending on the organ. Organs that require iodine in the pure form have enzymes that make iodine from iodide salt and will do this on their own. The breast tissue is one of these organs which do this. Iodine in pure unbound form does not occur anywhere in nature in any food source. All ingestible forms of iodine are in the iodide form. The enzyme which accomplishes this conversion in the thyroid gland is called thyroid peroxidase and the one in breast tissue is lacto peroxidase. Lugol's solution and some other supplements have both forms in it and some physicians have a belief that this is a more superior supplement than just potassium iodide because the body will use both forms without the need for any enzymatic conversion. Elemental iodine should be taken on an empty stomach about a half-hour before meals or an hour after meals. Iodide is already bound so you can take iodide with food. You can even test iodine symporter with an iodine loading test or you can just do a simple skin absorption test to see does your body absorbs and needs more iodine. Put Lugol's solution on the skin and wait for a couple of hours. If the solution is absorbed through the skin, you probably have an iodine deficiency. When you do a loading test, sufficiency is achieved when you take a 50 mg tablet and more than 90 percent of iodine is excreted in 24 hours of urine collected. If you are deficient in iodine and still have a high rate of excretion, it is a malfunction in sodium/iodide symporter. That is why you need to do both the spot test and the loading test to be sure. If you are prone to thyroid issues you must test your iodine levels and thyroid hormones to see if supplemental iodine is something you need. There were some studies that showed that some individuals are prone to developing subclinical hypothyroidism if supplemented with iodine, but again it is not iodine but malfunctioning of the thyroid that is a real problem and also in initial stages it can be a normal homeostatic response. Most of the people will have no issues and if you supplement with iodine and get subclinical hypothyroidism that is present for more than 6 months you might have a real disease in the future. I can compare it to prediabetes for example. It is not sugar that is the issue it is the malfunctioning of the body and it is not iodine that is an issue but malfunctioning of the body as well. In Japan, for example, they traditionally eat sea vegetables in a regular diet. They use kelp as a spice instead of table salt and also eat other types of algae in salads. The average intake of iodine for a Japanese woman is 13.8 mg a day. That is 13,800 mcg a day on average. Some studies have put this number lower to around 5 to 6 mg we do not have the exact number. However, there are no higher levels of subclinical hypothyroidism or other thyroid issues in Japan than anywhere else in the world. Japanese women, on the other hand, have very low rates of breast cancer and thyroid issues compared to western counterparts and this fact might have other contributing factors than just iodine but iodine itself is correlated. Average American will consume 200 mcg. RDA was set with the intention to prevent goiter only and as low as they can get away with.

The thyroid gland gets the first pick for iodine and that can leave the rest of the organs severely deficient. The reason why you would find recommendations from alternative doctors to take no more than 12.5 mg of iodine during pregnancy is because Japanese women have that level of intake. They want to protect themselves from liability in a case of complications during pregnancy. If you have deformed baby for example or something bad is happening, you would not be able to force any legal action against them because you will have to prove the correlation with iodine supplement and you will have to prove why that is not the case in Japan where women have even more iodine. Theoretically, you can take as much iodine as you want. There are for example 50 mg tablets that are designed to protect the population from radioactive iodine radiation exposure of the thyroid in the case of a nuclear emergency. Iodine Thyroid blocking is the technique used to stop or reduce the thyroid gland's ability to absorb inhaled or ingested radioiodine. There were concerns that some of the algae coming from Japan might be radioactive due to a Fukushima disaster. They were but by the time you will have them in stores radioactivity will be long gone. Radioiodine has a radioactive decay half-life of about eight days. When you take the iodine as a supplement at much higher levels than the recommended RDA during pregnancy if you don't have thyroid problems you will only have positive effects on the baby brain development. The only negative side effect is that iodine has an effect on baby brain alertness. You might have to deal with the fetus that is hyperactive after taking the supplement. The positive effect is that the average increase in IQ of the baby is estimated to be around 10 to 30 IQ points more than their parents. Iodine babies are much smarter than their non-supplemented brothers and sisters. On the other hand, a low level of iodine is associated with ADD later in life and a drop in IQ even if the baby does not suffer from blatant cretinism. Iodine is also needed during rapid brain development in the first three years after birth so you should be supplementing your baby as well. Also, it is needed for the development of the bones. Iodine deficiency can result in deformation of the skeletal structure such as dwarfism. In fossil records, endemic hypothyroidism typically is linked to specific ecological settings such as the high mountains regions where iodine is absent or occurs with very low concentrations in water and soil.

Imagine what can happen if someone is going to have a baby and don't supplement enough. The RDA recommendation is already miserable at 290 mcg for pregnant woman and if a woman has obesity or cardiovascular problems usually the doctor will take her off the salt so what would be the iodine intake if she is going to have a baby? There is no iodine added anywhere else except the table salt. It was added to the bread and milk but it was pulled out and only mandatory obligation now is to add it to the table salt. What happens when a cardiologist, for example, takes the woman of the salt before she gets pregnant and then from one specialist to another somehow, they all forget to tell her to supplement with iodine at an adequate level when she does get pregnant? Well, we would see an increase in ADD and a lowering of the IQ. From the year 2000 to 2006 the rate of ADD climbed 500 percent in the US. Health gurus that advocate to people to decrease salt intake and eat healthy for the sake of the baby will cause more damage if they do not know exactly what they are doing because taking off the salt in obese people is good and losing weight is good but only if you add sea vegetables or supplemental iodine to the diet. You take mother off the salt and you just have taken the baby out of iodine. Not knowing this can make your baby mentally retarded or in a mild form just hyperactive with ADD and lower IQ. Vegans are no exception. Around 80 percent of vegans are severely iodine deficient and around 90 percent of raw food vegans that are also low salt vegans at the same time are iodine deficient. Somehow no one had ever told them to add sea-green leafy vegetables into the diet. Algae are expensive but Lugol's solution is dirt cheap. Any pharmacy can make it. We need to eat marine plans on a daily basis or take supplemental iodine. That's the way it is. Our hominin ancestors had eaten sea vegetables and as a consequence, we have to eat them as well or we will have mentally retarded children. In Japan, they put seaweed in gummy bears and use kelp instead of salt. Kelp also has glutamate in it so it is a form of a substitute to MSG (monosodium glutamate).

When you saturate your body if you are a woman the maintenance will be around 6 mg just for thyroid function and around 5 mg for breast tissue and around 2 mg for the rest of the body per day. That is 13 mg just as maintenance. Men have lower estrogen and higher absorption rate and lower breast tissue (yes men have breast tissue and can also have breast tumor as well) so the daily requirements are much lower than this but still 10 times or even 20 times as proclaimed RDA value. And people need to ask the FDA why that is? Deficient thyroid and we are going to get enlargement with cysts and nodules and cancer, deficient breast and we are going to get breast cancer and inflamed tissue, cysts and nodules, lack of iodine to the ovaries and we are going to get cysts, nodules, pain (PCOS), inflammation, cancer, impotence, lack of iodine to the muscle and we are going to get pain, inflammation, fibrosis, weakness, and other symptoms of fibromyalgia. If you are a woman and have cysts in the breast tissue you have an iodine deficiency. Iodine is needed for the development of breast tissue and is excreted by mammary glands. There is four times iodine concentration in breast milk then in the thyroid gland. Iodine is very important for baby brain development. Iodine deficiency leads to the creation of cystic tissue (fluid-filled) and then leads to nodular tissue (becomes firm) and then leads to hyperplasia (the cellular division that is not normal) and then leads to cancer. Fibrocystic breast pain is iodine deficiency and muscle pain will disappear also with breast pain. Around 80 percent of fibromyalgia patients are iodine deficient and have a measurable decrease in pain when iodine deficiency is corrected. For 20 percent that don't, the cause of the pain is something else. It can be a herniated disk or something third. It will take from 3 to 6 months of iodine mega-dosing to improve cysts or nodules or disrupted glandular tissue. In severe cases, it might take even longer.

What usually happens when someone wants to add supplemental iodine to the diet just for health benefits and as breast cancer prevention or in times of pregnancy is that they might have some of the detoxifying effects of iodine and subclinical hypothyroidism in initial phases. For example, it might aggravate acne or give you diarrhea. Iodine is anti-mucolytic meaning it reduces mucus catarrh in both the intestines and the sinuses and the lungs. Iodine kills bacteria, viruses, and fungi everywhere including the lymph system and most of the lymph nodes are in the gut to fight off bad bacteria colony there. If you have an infection of some sort you might experience initial effects in the form of a Herxheimer's reaction (endotoxins released by the death of harmful microorganisms within the body resulting in a systemic inflammatory response) after iodine intake. Also, it will displace all of the other toxic halogens and that can lead to symptoms of detoxification or initial poisoning will be the more correct word. It also goes to the skin and acts the same. It is antiseptic and it kicks off halogens so for some people it might lead to initial acne breakout rashes or other skin reactions. Remember 20 percent of all iodine goes to the skin. If you are iodine deficient the body will use halogens instead of iodine and there will be a deposit of them instead of iodine. When iodine supplementation is initiated those halogens will be displaced and iodine will be used. Halogens are specific molecules in the straight line in the periodic table that are atomically similar to one another. The body has a hard time distinguishing between them. They are bromine, fluorine, iodine, and chlorine. You will drink fluoride in water if you live in countries that use that for water purification or if you don't drink fluoride you will drink chloride instead. Bromine is added to bakery products. Potassium bromate is a potent oxidizing agent that bleaches dough, improves its elasticity and creates thin bubbles inside as the bread rises. Potassium bromate is illegal in China, the European Union, Brazil, Canada, and most other countries. Bromine is associated with cancer in mice. In the US it has remained legal since it was first patented for use in baking bread, in 1914. First studies that showed that the body will pick up bromine instead of iodine and that will cause cancer in the thyroid and other organs have been done in 1982 in Japan. Iodine was used in the flour instead of bromine in the initial years but was removed because of the fears that it can cause hypothyroidism and was replaced with bromine. The way industry justifies this is that bromine will dissipate in high temperatures so the end product will have less than 20 parts per billion and that is considered safe. But this is not always the case and there is still fluoride in the water and chloride that are also iodine halogens. And then again bromine is added to soda pops, prescription drugs, automobile interior and fire retardants that you can breathe in and in many other products. Also, heavy metals like mercury and aluminum are chelates of iodine. They bound with each other. Consequently, iodine deficiency can cause heavy metal toxicity from aluminum and mercury. So exposure to aluminum, mercury, chlorine, fluorine, bromine all have negative effects on iodine metabolism within the body.

Dr. David Brownstein, author of the book "Iodine: Why You Need It / Why You Can't Live Without It", also has a thesis on how autoimmune thyroid diseases occur. To create energy in the body ATP, the body needs oxidative phosphorylation, the final stage of cellular respiration. A byproduct of this is hydrogen peroxide H2O2. Then H2O2 with TPO (thyroid peroxidase) oxidizes iodide to iodine. Thyroid peroxidase (TPO) is an enzyme that liberates iodine for addition onto tyrosine residues on thyroglobulin (TG) for the production of the thyroid hormones thyroxine (T4) or triiodothyronine (T3). When we consume potassium iodide it goes into the thyroid cells via sodium/iodide symporter and there it is converted to iodine thru oxidation. This process requires H2O2, TPO, NADPH activated by calcium and is inhibited by delta-iodolactone. In iodine deficiency, we do not have enough of delta-iodolactone. Delta-Iodolactone is an iodinated derivative of arachidonic acid with anti-cancer effects on diverse cancer cell lines (The role of iodine and delta-iodolactone in growth and apoptosis of malignant thyroid epithelial cells and breast cancer cells. Hormones (Athens). 2010 Jan-Mar;9(1):60-6). Also too little of delta-iodolactone and the body will not be able to stop oxidation of iodide. It regulates the oxidation of iodide. Then too much of the H2O2 will damage the TPO and if the body makes antibodies to the damaged TPO then that will worsen surrounding proteins such as thyroglobulin and then in the final stage the body will produce the antibodies to the damaged thyroglobulin and we will get Hashimoto disease. In Graves's disease, we will have anti-TSH antibodies. According to Dr. Brownstein, our bodies will only produce the optimal level of delta-iodolactone in a diet with 15mg of iodine a day and that is 100 times the current RDA. I could not find studies on this topic so it is not confirmed fact just speculation until more research is done. What is known for a fact is that selenium is part of glutathione peroxidase that the body uses to deactivate H2O2 and it is also a part of the enzyme called iodothyronine peroxidase that turns inactive T4 to active T3 thyroid hormone. Selenium deficiency will cause low glutathione peroxidase and inability to neutralize H2O2 and that will lead to damaging TPO and then to the Hashimoto disease. Also, low selenium is going to create low iodothyronine peroxidase and then low T3 level or in other words hypothyroid symptoms. Selenium is very important in all of this and we will understand why when we look at some studies later.

This is complicated biochemistry that is just in the research phase but still, many physicians have complete iodine phobia. Many healthcare professionals are scared of iodine because of the believe that iodine causes hypothyroidism. One of the reasons for this misconception is due to high TSH (Thyroid-stimulating hormone) levels in iodine therapy. It usually rises when there is hypothyroidism. However, as Dr. Brownstein explains:

"TSH has another function besides stimulating thyroid hormone production. It also helps to stimulate the body's production of the iodine transport molecules - the sodium-iodide symporter (NIS). Without adequate amounts of NIS, iodine would not be able to enter the cells and be utilized. Iodine-deficient patient's body does not require a large amount of NIS since there is little iodine that needs to be transported into the cells. However, when this individual begins to supplement with iodine, the extra iodine now needs to be transported into the cells. One way the body will accomplish this is to increase the production of TSH to stimulate more NIS... How long does TSH stay elevated? l have found that TSH may remain elevated for up to 6 months before lowering to normal. How high do TSH levels rise? The normal TSH level ranges from 0.5-4.5mlU/L. l have witnessed TSH levels elevated to 5-30mlU/L for a period of time sometimes up to six months before falling back to the normal range... The TSH will decline back to the reference range after the thyroid gland is saturated with iodine."

If you have a low iodine intake and all of us do, we need to supplement with iodine. If you have thyroid issues the best course of action is to consult the specialist and then decide what to do. Women who take too much supplemental iodine during pregnancy may give birth to babies with congenital hypothyroidism, a thyroid deficiency that, if left untreated, can lead to mental, growth, and heart problems and at the same time iodine deficiency is also typically suspected based on the development of goiter, hypothyroidism, or congenital hypothyroidism. Hypothyroidism is caused by iodine deficiency but taking iodine can shut down a thyroid and then also cause hypothyroidism or it might overstimulate the thyroid and you can end up with hyperthyroidism (extremely rare but it does happen sometimes). Nonetheless, the thyroid is just one of many organs in the body that needs it so if you have thyroid issues you still need iodine for other organs and that can be a problem. You need iodine for entire body functioning, not just thyroid so if you have thyroid issues you have a big problem. When you go to the licensed MD or specialists, they will have iodine phobia not because they are scared of iodine but because they are scared of lawsuits. They will conveniently forget that the entire body needs iodine not just thyroid and even if you have thyroid issues, they will give synthetic hormones or other drugs or surgery just so that they can avoid iodine. Here is for example what Mayo Clinic has to say about it: "It is true that iodine deficiency can cause hypothyroidism. But iodine deficiency is rare in the United States and other developed countries since the addition of iodine to salt (iodized salt) and other foods. If iodine deficiency isn't the cause of hypothyroidism, then iodine supplements provide no benefit and should not be used. In fact, for some people with abnormal thyroid glands, too much iodine can cause or worsen hypothyroidism. Hypothyroidism can be safely and effectively treated with the synthetic thyroid hormone levothyroxine (Synthroid, Levothroid, others)."

In medical schools and in practice the majority of the doctors learn that iodine supplementation will exaggerate already existing autoimmune (Hashimoto's) thyroiditis and this is true and backed by studies (The effect of iodine restriction on thyroid function in patients with hypothyroidism due to Hashimoto's thyroiditis. Yonsei Med J. 2003 Apr 30;44(2):227-35). Some even believe that iodine supplementation will create autoimmune (Hashimoto's) thyroiditis just by itself if there is a genetic predisposition. High levels of thyroid antibodies are associated with hypothyroidism symptoms therefore high levels of TPO antibodies and TSH levels are associated with progression of subclinical hypothyroidism to overt hypothyroidism. However, in some people, this will happen and in some, it won't. Some people even with Hashimoto's will have no aggravation with iodine and will even have a lessening of the disease. It was a big mystery that scientists contributed to individual genetic predisposition. But that was not correct and now we know why iodine aggravates Hashimoto's. The answer is selenium deficiency in most of the patients tested. Selenium deficiency is the underlying prerequisite for iodine-induced thyroid damage in Hashimoto's thyroiditis. In this study (Supplemental selenium alleviates the toxic effects of excessive iodine on thyroid. doi: 10.1007/s12011-010-8728-8) they observed that when selenium is supplemented along with iodine, TPO has returned to normal values. In a group that just had iodine TPO decreased but also it started to decrease with excess selenium intake. Therefore, the optimal levels of selenium alleviated the effects of iodine to TPO levels. This Chinese study (they have big problems with selenium depletion of the soil) showed that if iodine and selenium are increased together, no goiter will accrue and that resolved the whole mystery of Hashimoto's and iodine connection. In one more Chinese study (Selenium upregulates CD4(+) CD25(+) regulatory T cells in iodine-induced autoimmune thyroiditis model of NOD.H-2(h4) mice. Endocr J. 2010;57(7):595-601. Epub 2010 Apr 27) they concluded: "These data suggest that CD4(+) CD25(+) T cells play an important role in the development of AIT. Se supplementation may restore normal levels of CD4(+) CD25(+) T cells by up-regulating the expression of Foxp3 mRNA in mice with AIT." Now, this is a mouthful so let us decipher this language. AIT means autoimmune thyroiditis or Hashimoto's where our own immune system attacks the thyroid gland. Immune cells that do this are T cells of different types. Their regulation is done by expression of specific gene Foxp3 mRNA. That gene will stimulate the production of specific types of T cells CD4(+), CD25(+), that are known as TREG or Tregs, that have a suppressive effect on regular T cells. Tregs regulate and maintain self-tolerance by suppressing the response to self-antigens that all of us have and these self-attacking antigens do have a physiological function in the body in normal ranges. A deficit in Tregs cell numbers or function leads to autoimmune diseases (Foxp3+ CD25+ CD4+ natural regulatory T cells in dominant self-tolerance and autoimmune disease. Immunol Rev. 2006 Aug;212:8-27). The problem is created when the production of these auto-destructive T cells exceeds normal values and if there is no suppression of excessive amounts of them the disease will happen. They will attack the host and immune responses will be deleterious to the host creating autoimmune disease. What they did in the study is that they took healthy mice and then mega dosed them with iodine for eight weeks to create AIT. After eight weeks their AIT worsened dramatically. Then they separated that group into two and for the next eight weeks were supplementing selenium to one group of AIT induced mice. They gave them selenium in addition to iodine and the AIT returned to normal healthy state even though high-dose iodine had continued.

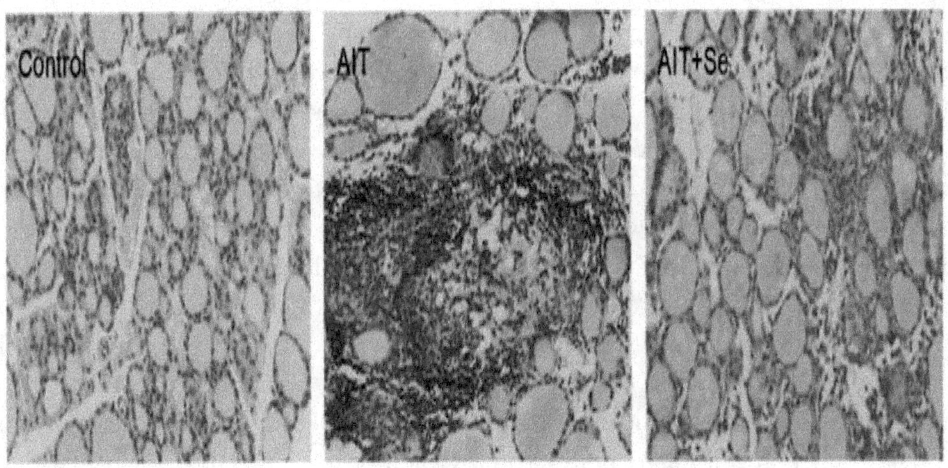

In the AIT group mice had dead tissue with enlarged cells and goiter. Thyroid weight doubled in the AIT group but returned to normal when supplemented with selenium. The thyroid shrank and the section that you can see in the image resembled a normal thyroid. In addition, CD4+CD25+Foxp3+ Tregs Cells were reduced by high iodine and TgAb antibodies were elevated but returned to normal after 8 weeks of selenium even though high iodine intake continued. The implication is that selenium-iodine balance may be needed to maintain proper Tregs cell populations and that selenium supplementation may restore normal regulation of autoimmunity. This is accepted now and this was not a single study but a series of them. Here is another one that was done in China with the same result (Effect of excessive iodine on immune function of lymphocytes and intervention with selenium. J Huazhong Univ Sci Technolog Med Sci. 2007 Aug;27(4):422-5). Why does selenium mitigate AIT? Like I wrote earlier besides maintaining proper Tregs cell populations selenium deficiency will cause low glutathione peroxidase and then that will cause the inability to neutralize H2O2 and then that will lead to damaging TPO and then to the Hashimoto disease. At the same time, low selenium is going to create low iodothyronine peroxidase and then low T3 level or in other words hypothyroid symptoms. If you take selenium as a healthy thing to do but at the same time you do not "megadose" with iodine but continue to get 150 to 200 mcg/day recommended RDA, bad things are going to happen as well. This study was done on the population in the north of the Zaire where extremely high levels of cretinism is present due to the iodine deficiency and at the same time, they have severe selenium deficiency as well (Selenium deficiency mitigates hypothyroxinemia in iodine-deficient subjects. doi: 10.1093/ajcn/57.2.271S). They didn't give the subjects iodine, just selenium. Because of the selenium deficiency, the glutathione peroxidase activity was low and hydrogen peroxide produced during thyroid hormone synthesis aggravated hypothyroidism by stimulating thyroxin metabolism. Selenium supplementation was given without the "mega-dosing" of iodine. In the study cretins and schoolchildren were just supplemented for 2 months with a normal average dose of selenium of 50 mcg of selenium per day in the form of selenomethionine. Only one Brazil nut contains selenium in the range from 68-91 mcg depending on the size of the nut. An optimal dose of daily selenium for adult individuals is from 200 to 400 mcg/day depending on weight. After 2 months of 50 mcg/day of selenium supplementation, the substantial reduction in serum T4 in virtually every subject happened. In schoolchildren, serum free thyroxin (fT4) decreased from 11.8 nmol/L to 8.4 nmol/L and serum reverse triiodothyronine (rT3) decreased from 12.4 nmol/L to 9.0 nmol/L on average while mean serum T3 and mean TSH remained stable. There is a range of similar studies with the same conclusion (Effect of selenium supplementation on thyroid hormone metabolism in an iodine and selenium deficient population. Clin Endocrinol (Oxf). 1992 Jun;36(6):579-83). Iodine without selenium can create hypothyroidism, so too can selenium without iodine. Both are needed.

Do your own research, consult a specialist, do blood testing and decide what you are going to do. You can start with a low level of supplemental iodine and selenium and then test to see the levels of thyroid hormones. If everything is in the normal range, then increase the dose and test and if everything is a fine increase again and test. If you get subclinical hypo or hyperthyroidism, then stay on that level for a couple of months and test to see if the thyroid is back to normal. If not, you might have an autoimmune disease. When you take an iodine supplement and have an increase in thyroid-stimulating hormone (TSH) that will be diagnosed as hypothyroidism but it is not no matter what MD is telling you he is wrong. Elevated TSH without lowering of T3 or T4 or clinical signs of hypothyroidism such as fatigue and hair loss is not hypothyroidism. It is increased TSH because TSH stimulates not just thyroid but also iodine transport enzymes for the rest of the body or in other words sodium-iodide symporter (NIS) responsible for allowing the iodine to enter the cells. For all of the MD's out there that are going to read this or if they ask you tell them this. More iodine means more TSH, more TSH means more NIS created, more NIS created means more iodine transported to the cells and thyroid gland. It could take to 6 months after starting the supplementation for the TSH to normalize. MD's that do this in their practice have reported that normal TSH range of 0.5-4.5mIU/l usually goes to 5-30mIU/L for periods within 6 months of iodine treatment before coming down to normal. It is a normal response and you don't have to freak out because of it. MD will usually freak out because he has a lawsuit on his mind.

The problem is that even if you do have the issues with thyroid you still need iodine for the rest of the body. So even if you need to avoid iodine because of the thyroid you still need to take iodine for other tissues and immune system. Thank our hominin ancestors for that. You can try another approach and that is to shut down thyroid with mega-dosing to saturate the rest of the body in a short period of time. We need 1,500 mg of iodine for full saturation so you might take for example 100 mg a day every morning like in the case of nuclear emergencies. In this case, you will want the supplement that has both types of iodine and iodide in there to eliminate the need for any conversion within the body. The body will not be able to convert all of this mega-dosed iodide to iodine so you will need the supplement that has both like Lugol's solution and not just potassium iodide but again all of that iodine might not get utilized fully. Long term steady approach will give you in my opinion better result but this mega dosing for saturation might work also. I don't really know. You can mega dose quickly to get it done and then after 15 days you can go back to maintenance and after a month or two test the levels of thyroid hormones. If everything is ok, then you can continue with maintenance for the rest of your life. Or you might have iodine phobia and avoid it completely, it is your choice. If you are already taking thyroid hormone and you are iodine deficient you can start the iodine supplementation and if hyperthyroid symptoms occur, you will lower the medication and if symptoms remain you can stop to take the medication completely. If not and your thyroid levels remain the same you will have to continue to take the medication. There is only one contraindication with supplementing with iodine that is real and that I know about. That is if you have hot nodules (nodules that produce excess thyroid hormone) in the thyroid gland. You will have to surgically remove them before iodine supplementation or they will be overstimulated causing hyperthyroidism and there is no cure for them only surgical removal.

It is important to remember that nothing in the body works in an isolated environment so most of the tests will be incomplete just by itself because they will not be able to pinpoint the root cause of the problem. If the thyroid gland does not work properly it might be the thyroid itself but it might not be. It depends. What tells the thyroid to produce hormones? It is a pituitary gland that spits out TSH that then tells the thyroid to work. What tells the pituitary to work? The answer is the hypothalamus. What tells the hypothalamus to work? The answer is the rest of the body. Hypothalamus is connected to the spinal cord and with all of the spinal cord sensors in the rest of the body. These sensors constantly analyze the condition of the body to see what the environment is. For example, when you have inflammation due to the bad diet and toxicity your body will respond by creating cortisol. Cortisol is the greatest anti-inflammatory known to medicine. When some health gurus preach about lowering cortisol it is complete nonsense. It is not the cortisol that is a problem. It is inflammation and toxicity that will force the body to react in a defensive manner to lower the stress in the form of inflammation. Cortisol is produced by adrenals and adrenals are one of the most important endocrine organs in the body. They produce cortisol, epinephrine, and many other hormones but the cortisol itself will have an effect on lowering the production of TSH. Any inflammation in the body will raise the cortisol and then that will lower TSH and thyroid function will be decreased. The thyroid works directly with adrenal glands and if one is up the other will be down.

There is one more biological action of iodine that I want to mention. Iodine plays a role in histamine metabolism. Histamine is a protein that is present in all cells in the body and has a role in healing by triggering a pro-inflammatory response. For example, when we have allergic reaction histamine is involved and the usual treatment for allergies is anti-histaminic drug regimen. There is a whole list of histamine release symptoms depending on the location on where is it released. For example, you can have an allergic reaction in the stomach and that will cause cramping pain and diarrhea or have allergic rhinitis if there is an irritant in the air. Histamine is also released independently from allergic reactions. If histamine that is released fails to break down, there will be histamine intolerance. There is an enzyme named diamino oxidase that will neutralize histamine. Problem is that besides normal histamine release in the body there is also histamine present in the food and when this enzyme does not function properly there can be a buildup of histamine that will cause histamine pro-inflammatory reactions in the body. These reactions depend on the place where histamine is reacting or in other words, it depends on histamine receptors that are triggered. There are four different receptors that are present everywhere from skin, uterus, cardiovascular system, gastrointestinal system, respiratory tract, bone marrow, and central nervous system. One day it can give you skin rash, another day panic attack with insomnia, third day nausea, fourth day painful menstrual periods and so on. The list is endless. The problem is that iodine is used inside the body to decrease the levels of histamine. Iodine inhibits the conversion of histidine to histamine (The degradation reaction of histidine with iodine; doi.org/10.1002/recl.19670860406) and stops the histamine release (The suppressive mechanism of histamine release from rat peritoneal mast cells of iodine-enriched eggs. Int J Tissue React. 2001;23(3):73-9). Mast cells are one of the primary cells in the body that create histamine. The things that can go wrong in the body if there is iodine deficiency is the never-ending story of cascading effects. You can combine all of the symptoms of hypothyroidism with all of the symptoms of the rest of the body iodine deficiency issues, not just thyroid and then you can add a list of the symptoms of histamine intolerance and take your pick. But again it is important that you do not do medical intervention just by yourself. Every mineral has an opposite mineral so taking an excess of one in the supplemental form will create a deficiency of opposite mineral. That is why it is important to eat complete mineral-rich foods and let the body do the process of mineral balancing.

However, that is not possible anymore due to soil erosion and mineral depletion. On top of that, we have shifted from a plant-based diet to animal products based diet. If you eat animal products, refined processed foods with sugar and oil and regular mineral-depleted commercially grown plant foods, you are in a problem. It is almost certain that you will be magnesium deficient and also iodine deficient and also trace and rare mineral deficient. At the same time, you probably are going to have toxic levels of iron and excessive levels of calcium. But before you do any change do your own research and consult the licensed specialist that has a good reputation in this area of expertise. What you should do is to track everything you eat in charts for a month and then analyze your diet nutrition profile. You will have the insight on what minerals you need. For example, 98 percent of Americans have potassium deficiency due to excessive sodium intake but lowering sodium intake will worsen iodine deficiency. If you want to take a mineral supplement you should only take iodine because it is bioavailable and never take any metallic mineral in a pill form. Trace and rare-earth minerals are the ones that are hardest to supplement. At present day there are some supplements that are made from organic matter, usually expensive and not potent enough to make a real difference but they will have real organic minerals in them and all of them including rare-earth minerals. They are created from plant-based biomass suspended in an unaltered ionic solution and in the ratios naturally found within the original humate/lignite source. Fulvic Acid is the substance found in humus and is created in extremely small amounts by millions of beneficial microbes that work on the decaying plant matter. It combines with a range of minerals to create a complex molecular compound. Fulvic Acid molecule is capable of binding to 65 or more organic minerals and trace elements. Fulvic Acid and different microbes in the soil work to activate the nutrients within decomposing biomass in the soil so that they can be utilized by the cells of plants. If there is a biomass and it is clear from pollution then it can be used as an organic mineral solution for human consumption as a concentrated, all-natural plant-based source of over 70 ionic minerals. There are some other supplements, for example, the famous Shilajit. Shilajit (Sanskrit: शिलाजतु, śilājatu, Salajit in Urdu) or Mumijo. A thick, sticky tar-like substance that was first known mineral supplement in the history of herbal medicine and it is one of the oldest substances ever used in Ayurveda medicine. It is used in Ayurveda and Unani, the traditional Indian system of medicine for thousands of years with a first recorded use in the sixth century BCE. It has been reported to contain at least 85 minerals in ionic form, as well as triterpenes, humic acids, and fulvic acid. In modern times there is also a process of extracting trace minerals from sea salt and creating trace mineral compound known as ORMUS. ORMUS is usually just used as a fertilizer but some people will take it directly as a supplement and I don't recommend this. The best course of action will be to correct your diet with organic high-quality diet but that will be hard to obtain if you don't have your own garden and do mineral enrichment of the soil with biomass or ORMUS yourself. Even organically grown food today is depleted to some extent. Some produce will have most of the minerals that they should have if the plant has a big and deep root system like walnuts or Brazil nuts. Regular fruit also will have a root system that goes deeper to the ground but every other crop that is grown on annual bases is completely depleted. Grains, vegetables, seeds, beans all of them are mineral depleted. Only perennial plants with deep and big root systems will have full nutritional value and organically grown food. Most of us living today take prescription drugs for all of our illnesses but we do not have a drug deficiency. We have nutrient deficiency.